Daniel Callahan

*Why America's Quest
for Perfect Health
Is a Recipe for Failure*

SIMON & SCHUSTER

False
Hopes

SIMON & SCHUSTER
Rockefeller Center
1230 Avenue of the Americas
New York, NY 10020

Copyright © 1998 by Daniel Callahan
All rights reserved,
including the right of reproduction
in whole or in part in any form.
SIMON & SCHUSTER and colophon are
registered trademarks of Simon & Schuster Inc.
Designed by Edith Fowler
Manufactured in the United States of America

10   9   8   7   6   5   4   3   2   1

Library of Congress Cataloging-in-Publication Data

Callahan, Daniel, date.
    False hopes : why America's quest for perfect
health is a recipe for failure /
Daniel Callahan.
        p.   cm.
    Includes bibliographical references and index.
    1. Medical care—United States.   2. Medicine—
Philosophy.   I. Title.
RA395.A3C322   1998
362.1'0973—dc21   97-40541   CIP
ISBN 0-684-81109-X

Acknowledgments

I confess that I'm never eager to read other people's draft papers, much less their book manuscripts. But I rarely admit that to those who ask me to do so; and I usually do it. In a general conspiracy of silence, it may well be that none of us like to read each other's drafts, which means that some readers of this manuscript may have suffered in silence also, saying yes to my request when they would have preferred to say no.

Yet perhaps I should hesitate about attributing to others what I sometimes feel. I was once told that a friend felt hurt that I had not asked him to read a draft of an earlier book. Since he had read the draft of a still earlier book, I had deliberately decided to spare him another request. All I can say is that I apologize to that one other person in a thousand (million?) who might be hurt that I did not ask for help. Next time.

As for those who did act as readers, let it be recorded that I consider such work hard. But it is not thankless, and the many comments I received have made this book much better than it otherwise would have been. Those readers include Sissela Bok, George Annas, Courtney Campbell, Anthony Robbins, Kenneth Schaffner, Bryan Norton, Paul Menzel, Joy Mappes, Mark Sagoff, Bette Crigger, Bruce Jennings, and Erik

7

ACKNOWLEDGMENTS

Parens. Dorothy Rice provided me with much help on the question of the compression of morbidity, and Jennifer Stuber worked her research wonders many times on many subjects. Ellen McAvoy, who has helped me with almost all of my books, corrected the too many drafts, and I am both grateful and apologetic. Dan Fox, president of the Milbank Fund, was an early and most timely supporter of this book.

Contents

Preface

When I began this book during the hopeful days of 1994, there was every expectation that the United States would imminently have a universal health insurance plan. How could it be otherwise? Everyone seemed to want one, and with good reason. Some 37 million people lacked health insurance, millions more lived with daily threats to their coverage, public opinion was supportive, Bill Clinton had campaigned for it, and corporate America was looking for a way out from under rising health care costs. Moreover—we optimists felt—if the Clinton plan didn't make it, there were enough other schemes in the congressional wings to guarantee at least something. It was not, then, a matter of whether, but of how and what. Surely *something*.

Surely nothing, it turned out. No plan made it through Congress then—not a single bill, not a single reform. By 1997, the 37 million uninsured had grown to 41 million and only one other bill had been passed; the two presidential candidates in 1996 had all but ignored the issue (save for insisting that they had a pain-free way to save Medicare)—and 34 percent of Americans polled thought the health care system had become worse over the past few years.[1] Projections for the future of the Medicare Trust Fund, of crucial importance for the elderly, showed bankruptcy by 2001 or shortly thereafter and enormous deficits in the following decades.

For a time there was considerable optimism that managed care could tame the constant annual increase in health care costs, and it seemed to do so in 1995–1996. But by early 1997, upward pressure had appeared here and there once again.[2] That has been cold water on hot enthusiasm. For if no universal coverage came out of the 1994 Clinton push, the President's proposal inadvertently galvanized the private sector. That sector turned to managed care, partly as a defense against a possible Clinton success in establishing centralized cost controls, and partly as an innovative way to increase market competition, organize health care more efficiently, and give the private sector a leg up on government. The return of cost increases is sobering.

All these developments were important, but they were not the only ones catching my eye during the early 1990s. I was also drawn to the mounting evidence that not just the United States, but *every* nation was undergoing some degree of stress in managing and paying for its health care system — regardless of how that system was structured and financed. Schemes that were thought to spell salvation in the United States were running up against problems elsewhere; most prominently and disturbingly, universal health care was troubled. No country, it turns out, seems to have a handle on the best way to reform its health care system to keep pace with an aging population, unsettled economic conditions, technological progress, and public demand. Reform was on every country's agenda. It had to be. Modern medicine is too expensive to be ignored. It is increasingly too expensive to be viable.

In 1993, the World Bank issued an important report, *Investing in Health*, which pointed out the continuing gap in health status between rich and poor nations.[3] It also noted that many poor nations were making the epidemiological transition (as it is called) from rates and causes of death characteristic of them — mainly infectious disease — to the kinds of death and sickness rates once typical of affluent countries, principally chronic disease. This transition was surely a sign of progress, but it was by no means clear how still-struggling countries could pay for the new, more modern medical techniques and demands being heaped upon them. The World Health Organization (WHO), which had for two decades pressed for a strengthening and expansion of primary care services in the developing countries, was forced, by the middle of the decade, to reinvigorate a drive that had partially stalled.[4] In China and Southeast Asia, and in much of Central and Eastern Europe — once the home of universal, if poorly financed and often corrupt, care systems — privatization and a turn to the market became the new gospel, as they did also for many countries in Latin America.

Most unsettling, perhaps, have been the changes creeping insistently through Western Europe. Those countries — still the showcase of popular and well-managed health care systems equitably accessible to all — have begun to show the first loose threads from an unraveling of the post–World War II welfare state. Their systems, beset with rising costs, are high on the budgetary hit lists of political leaders. Europe, too, is now looking to the market and reduced public benefits for its own future, even if not quite so intensively as parts of Asia and Latin America. In one of the odder twists, a number of Western European countries have been intently watching some American developments, particularly the health care priority-setting of the Oregon Medicaid program and the organization and spread of managed care. It is surely a sign of an unsettled health care universe when other countries, with historically far less expensive, equally effective, more popular systems, look to the United States for ideas — to us, who have led the world in devising the most expensive, least equitable system of all. But our own anxiety has generated some interesting experiments, and they attract attention.

It is, then, the universality of the reform drive that seems to me important, particularly the global casting about for solutions that has come to mark our era. If everyone is having a problem, and all are looking for answers, this suggests a more basic issue than is ordinarily entertained by those responsible for reform. As I began thinking about this possibility, an obvious—but little-examined—fact stared me in the face: almost all the reform efforts, in the United States and elsewhere, assume that the solution to the health care problem lies in better organization and financing. But I wondered if that "solution" was addressing the real problem. I began entertaining an alternative idea. Perhaps it is the very values of modern medicine, its most cherished and celebrated aims and commitments, that are beginning to give us trouble. Perhaps we must reexamine those values, and change some of them, before we can have any hope of devising health care systems that can successfully endure into the future.

I was especially struck by a common thread in the various national struggles: no matter how much money is spent, and no matter what the health gains, they never seem enough. Could it be that in modern medicine we have devised a set of medical aspirations and practices that guarantee health system stress and perhaps, in some cases, eventual collapse? And which no less guarantee that, whatever progress is made, it will always seem insufficient to meet the "needs" of the day—needs that are constantly being refined and upgraded precisely because of the improvements in health care and ongoing medical progress? Those are the general questions I have come to pursue.

In 1992, I was able to initiate an international project at The Hastings Center: "The Goals of Medicine: Setting New Priorities." The project included working research groups in fourteen different countries and, over a four-year period, tried to address the most basic questions about the appropriate ends of medicine.[5] This book represents a parallel project, taking many of the themes of the "Goals" research and tying them to a long-standing interest in the nature and future of medicine. And my following of environmental debates suggested to me the central theme for this book: the need for a view of medicine that would be at once equitable and sustainable. The problem is a present model of medicine that is, for all its excitement, increasingly and painfully unaffordable. Just as we need a sustainable environment, we need a sustainable medicine.

I also became aware that, in wanting to ask a different set of questions about the reform of health care—substantive questions, not simply financial and policy questions—I was part of a mainly unsung tradition of medical reform that has appeared over the past few decades. While most reform efforts focus on technical, administrative, and economic changes, the tradition I have in mind has worried about the models, visions, and broad aims that have animated health care systems, and about how to set fresh ones in place of those whose time has passed. The 1960s and 1970s saw the first real outburst from those writing in this vein, and it became clear as I reread those works (only some of which I had read at the time) that I am one more person in the recent line of those trying to get us to think differently about the nature of medicine and health, not just about health care systems and their financing.

The contemporary pioneer of this tradition was the biologist René Dubos, whose 1954 book *Mirage of Health* called into question the then imminently anticipated total conquest of disease. It would not happen, he said, not soon, not ever.[6] The theologian Ivan Illich attracted attention in 1976 with *Medical Nemesis*, a book that blamed doctors (excessively) for their alleged stranglehold on health care and for their supposed brainwashing of patients to do their bidding.[7] In the 1970s, Illich, the British physician John Powles, an American lawyer, Rick Carlson, and a British professor of social medicine, Thomas McKeown, each showed in a systematic way that there is no clear correlation between population health and medical care.[8] Carlson boldly predicted "the end of medicine," by which he meant the gradual recognition of the diminishing impact of physicians and hospitals on health, which he expected to become all the more salient by the year 2000. And so, in some ways—but not others—it has.

While there has surely been a decline in the number of hospital beds over the past two decades—a tribute to the recognition of an expensive excess of beds and to a more vigorous use of outpatient surgery and other medical procedures—the role of doctors has remained strong; and their role in prevention, not just cure and amelioration, has been more strongly emphasized. Carlson and Illich espoused a deprofessionalization and deregulation of medicine, to induce people to be more responsible for their own health and to be free to pursue that health as they saw fit. Deprofessionalization has not yet occurred, at least within mainline health care. On the contrary, the outcome assessment movement, seeking to evaluate the effectiveness of medical technologies and therapies, has emphasized scientifically informed professional judgment—even as there is, side by side with it, a burgeoning self-help and alternative-medicine movement. *Pace* Ivan Illich, it seems that patients and physicians share most of the same goals; it is thus a mistake to see the former as dupes of the latter, even if one grants the undoubted sway of physicians.

An enduring contribution by Rick Carlson was his astute analysis of five approaches to health: (1) a fatalism that assumes health is beyond human control and in the hands of the gods; (2) the public health approach, with its stress on disease prevention in the context of the health of populations and intervention into the social and environmental order; (3) a prevention approach focused on individuals rather than populations (as now pursued by HMOs); (4) an emphasis on "the natural," stressing the self-limiting character of disease and the role of the individual in pursuing health; and (5) the pursuit of health through

18

services provided by a medical care system organized to treat the symptoms and causes of disease when and as they appear.[9] As will become clear, it is the second and fourth strategies that have most attracted me, just as they most attracted many of the writers in the reform tradition I identified above just before and after the 1970s.[10]

Yet while there are some clear family resemblances between what I want to say and what those who precede me in this "tradition" have said, there are also some differences. Recent evidence strengthens the earlier claim that there is no significant correlation between population health status and medical care, even as it shows that among some groups (notably the elderly), medical care improves health. But the earlier group of writers did not focus, as I will, quite so much on the ideals and aims of modern medicine, much less the idea of progress. In looking for a sustainable medicine, I am searching for a medicine that learns how to stop growing, how to stop consuming ever more resources, how to find some finite goals, and then how to stop once they have been achieved. I don't believe that note was struck earlier. It also seems clear now that if health promotion and disease prevention, at present much championed, are ever to achieve parity with acute-care medicine, we must be prepared to rethink today's medical priorities to make the potential gains in health status efficacious. More generally, a serious transformation will require *taking money away* from the acute-care sector, including research into the cure of many lethal diseases, and using it instead for prevention research and massive educational efforts designed to change health-related behavior.

I am indebted, in any event, to those who began developing the idea of a basic shift in medical thinking. As they surely discovered, trying to change modern scientific medicine and its health care offspring is like trying to shift and channel glaciers. But the effort is worth making, and if one generation fails then another should take up the task. From time to time glaciers do change course, usually because of great environmental and climatic changes. Those of us who look to decisive changes in thinking about medicine—someday or other—can only hope that their ideas will come at a historical moment when the social environment is ripe for them. That every nation is now feeling the economic pinch, and many the pincers, of trying to live out the expansive, insupportable dream of modern medicine may provide that moment.

A more personal word is also in order. In three of my earlier books, the question of medicine's stance toward mortality preoccupied me. In *Setting Limits: Medical Goals in an Aging Society*, I explored how we might think about aging and the provision of health care. In *What Kind of Life: The Limits of Medical Progress*, I took up the problem of resource allocation; and in *The Troubled Dream of Life: In Search of a Peaceful Death*, I probed our cultural stance toward death. Those issues are still on my mind, and echoes of them will be heard in this book. Getting older myself, feeling death scratching at my door with his scythe, and fretting about expensive medical bills do little to push them aside. But I am much more concerned here in moving to a new plane, where the possibilities and limits of medicine confront our seemingly insatiable appetite for more and better life. I am edgy, I confess, about using the term "sustainable," a word that is a little too chic, a little too vague, a little too familiar. But no better term appeared.

Should we change our understanding of medicine, or should we change our understanding of life? I suspect we have to do both, and somehow or other do them at the same time. A life dependent on medical props and progress for its meaning seems to me not a life at all, even if our body keeps going for a time. A medicine that must forever promise new miracles, new bodies, and new selves to get its research supported and justify its big money strikes me as a medicine that has lost its way, forgetting that it is not the key to the good life.

In trying to advance a more modest agenda for medicine, I am also advancing a view of human life—restrained, perhaps, but not despairing, not without hope of its own kind. While I do not here want to repeat the argument of *The Troubled Dream of Life*, I can briefly summarize it. Death is an inescapable reality of human life and always will be. Medicine must build that understanding into its mission, not seek to overcome it. Our humanity is, in great part, defined by our willingness to accept and live with death. Modern scientific medicine has been unwilling to do so, which is why it has been so much easier to find money to search for a cure for cancer than to find money for better palliative and home care for those with terminal cancer.

Of course death, and the illnesses leading to it, are not easily accepted. Hope has always been important in medicine, right back to Hippocrates nearly 2,500 years ago, and it remains important today, whether for the doctor and patient struggling with a serious illness, or for biomedical researchers trying to know more and do better. But we have come to make our hope depend on the delusion that medicine can, through research and refined clinical skills, master death and illness and, as a managerial aside, do so with some respectable cost-benefit ratio. That hope has sustained twentieth-century medicine. It is the wrong hope. A decent, fulfilled life for the individual does not require it, and for society to pursue it is folly. The issues I want to talk about in this book are not easy to think or talk about; many of them may make us nervous. But I have come to believe that, if we can work through some of them, we might lay the foundation stone for a more satisfying understanding of life and medicine than the one we have lived with for some decades now. We might even take comfort in the thought that there are ways of living with medicine, and living with ourselves, that do not require the constant pushing of the envelope of medical possibility that is our present lot.

If this book reflects an underlying view of death and its

place in a human life, it also reflects a view of the expenditure of public and private money to combat sickness, to improve health, and to defer death. Again, while I do not want to summarize the thesis of *What Kind of Life*, this much is worth repeating to make clear my own biases and inclinations: health care is only one of many valuable ways to spend our money, and a good society is one that tries to find an appropriate place for the improvement of health, neither neglecting it (as some countries have done) nor allowing it to trump other important needs (as has been the American proclivity; we spend more per capita on health care than any other nation). I do not think our nation can afford to keep pursuing medical and health improvement as intensely as we have done over the past fifty years. Perfection has been the implicit aim, and it cannot be had.

I resist in particular the belief that the way to fiscal utopia is constant technological innovation. That seems to me an act of faith, nothing more. I do not share that faith. I may well be wrong. If so, I suppose I will line up as eagerly as the next person for any innovation that will help me. We shall see. I would also note that, by invoking throughout the book the ancient Greek tradition of *hygeia*—the notion that the body can take care of itself if helped to do so—I am not struggling against medicine itself but against the distortions introduced by a scientific medicine that has often forgotten some of the strengths of older traditions and practices.

A word is in order about the scope of this book. I have not tried to develop all the policy implications of my general thesis, much less to produce a policy blueprint. While the old axiom "The devil is in the details" is surely true, I have not myself worked out all the details in this case; more hands than I have would be needed. More important, I am trying to change the *nature* of the discussion about medicine, its goals, and its values: to see if we can find a fresh general picture to entertain in our minds, a different range of models, an alternative set of underlying values. Too often, in our practical American way, we neglect foundational and value issues, either taking them for granted and not examining them at all, or pushing them aside in our eagerness to get on with the immediate work. But it is just those issues that are the point of this book. Nonetheless, in an attempt to take the via media, I have also tried, toward the end of each chapter, to sketch out the policy implications of my analysis. I hope that will be sufficient.

I have a long way to go to make my thesis plausible, to find a way to an affordable, sustainable, equitable medicine. The first part of the book tries to lay out the foundation of a sustainable medicine, while the second part examines what it would take to build upon it. I begin by setting the thesis I want to develop, arguing in Chapter 1 the need for a sustainable, steady-state medicine. In Chapter 2, I show why the dream of modern medicine—with its roots in the idea of progress—ought now to be abandoned, and I show the price we pay for not giving up the dream. In Chapter 3, I take on that demigod, technological innovation—the most common means of fulfilling the idea of medical progress—and ask whether it can do for us what is claimed in its name. Medicine has developed a characteristic stance toward nature, and in Chapter 4, I explore and offer some antidotes to the kinds of poison that stance has introduced. I then examine, in Chapter 5, the modern medical response to suffering and the self, locating that response in modernism, whose problems it shares.

The next three chapters are a working out of some policy implications of what I propose. Chapter 6 focuses on the combination of public health (with its population-health orientation) and personal responsibility for health (with its individualistic perspective). Chapter 7 takes on the question of medicine and the market, asking what we are to make of the developing marriage between two utterly dissimilar ways of looking at human life and behavior. I take the confrontation between public-health and market perspectives to be fateful for the future of medicine. In Chapter 8, I examine the prospects for an equitable medicine if a sustainable medicine could carry the day. Chapter 9 saves the hardest problem for last: whether the modern (or postmodern, or postpostmodern) world, ever in search of hope, could ever come to accept a sustainable and steady-state medicine, which is psychologically most demanding even if most sensible.

CHAPTER ONE

Creating a
Sustainable Medicine

Every dream must end, even—perhaps especially—that of modern medicine. The dreams we have in our sleep cease when we awaken. They are gone whether we like it or not. Not so those fantasies we have invented in our waking lives. Since they project a better life, a more perfect world, they are not so easy to let go. The dream of modern medicine—that life, death, and illness can be scientifically dominated and pacified—will be one of the most difficult to give up. It has had us in its grip for at least two hundred years, and it has been remarkably satisfying in many respects. It has saved lives, eradicated many diseases, and relieved much suffering. It has been fueled by the seemingly reasonable conviction that, if we take up arms against a hostile nature, our ancient enemies—sickness, disability, and disease— can be overcome.

The fulfillment of that dream, it is said, requires only good and zealous science, wise patience, ample research money, and public support. Since none of us looks forward to disease and death, as a public we could hardly fail to support a dream so much in our own interest. By its deliverances, science has managed steadily to reinforce those interests.

How, then, when the dream is still so alive, even flourishing, can I contend that we must bring it to an end? And if it can be brought to a close, is there something better to put in its place—a dream that is more realistic, more plausible, and no less satisfying and hopeful? My short answer to these two questions is this: The dream of modern medicine is no longer viable as it stands. Even if unlimited resources were available, modern medicine cannot deliver on its most extravagant promises, nor even on many that seem modest and plausible. It cannot conquer infectious disease, and it will also fail in the foreseeable future to rid our lives of the main chronic killer diseases—cancer, heart disease, and stroke. Even if it succeeded in doing so, other lethal diseases would take their place on the top of the fatality lists. Not only do we not get out of this world alive, but except in case of accident we do not get out of it by any other route than a final, fatal disease.

What can be put in place of the impossible dream of medicine? My contention is that modern societies, beginning with our own, need a "sustainable" medicine, a term I borrow from the environmental movement. By it I mean a medicine that, in both research and health care delivery, aims for a steady-state plateau, at a level that is economically affordable and equitably available, and also at a level that is no less psychologically sustainable, satisfying most—but, of necessity, not all—reasonable health needs and expectations. I am after a change in the *ideals* and *hopes* of medicine, not simply in the way we organize and deploy the provision of care to sick people.

Toward a Third Era of Medicine

Medicine has gone through two great eras. The dividing line between them was the insight that the application of the scientific method could transform the mission and success of medicine. The first era of medicine was prescientific. Beyond some primitive observations and poorly based explanations (that of an imbalance of the four humors, for instance), there was not much that medicine could do for the sick and the dying. It could offer a little diagnosis, some degree of palliation and comfort, and, through a sharp eye for the psychological and spiritual needs of the ill, some shrewd ways of keeping hope alive in the face of the inevitable.

During this long era of human history (still extant in some poor areas of the world), the ideal of the physician's exclusive devotion to the welfare of the patient was formed (nurtured in the West by the Hippocratic tradition), and with that devotion the moral requirement of sensitivity and compassion. Hardly less important was the cultural and societal response to sickness and death. Every culture developed characteristic ways of giving meaning to, and making some sense of, the fact that human beings live with the constant threat of bodily destruction and death, and of mental disintegration and emotional chaos. Ritual patterns of response, usually religious, were brought to bear, and people were thereby helped to sustain a life in the midst of constant threats of extinction.

In its first era medicine did not wholly lack an idea of progress, but the notion was of a casual and random force—a little improvement here and a little there, over the centuries—not of great and dominating power. "Progress" was not a transforming vision of medical possibilities, nor were societal institutions and attitudes available to give it vitality. Resignation and acceptance of the human lot were the reigning values.

27

The second era of medicine might conveniently be dated from the writings of Francis Bacon in the early seventeenth century. In them lay the ideas, clear and unmistakable, that science provided the key to medical advancement, and that high on the agenda of a new medicine should be the aim of saving and extending life. There gradually followed, during the eighteenth and nineteenth centuries, the great early modern stream of gathering medical knowledge. Edwin Chadwick and the English sanitation movement, Pasteur and the germ theory of disease, Claude Bernard and the idea of the body as an integrated whole are only a few of many possible examples. Our era, into the twentieth century, has been marked by a faith in science and medical progress unabated to this day.

World War II and the decades just after it marked another great leap forward, as the pace of medical discovery and clinical application quickened and the dream of unlimited medical advances spread to the general public. The medical marketplace grew quickly as well during those years, a growth signaled by a great upswing in the cost of health care, now a highly valued commodity, and by the emergence of a massive medical-industrial complex devoted to turning medical progress and popular demand into large shareholder profits. By the 1960s in most developed countries the old prewar medicine had faded into the past, replaced by a different spirit, pace, and set of ambitions. The second era of medicine had hit its full stride, and we continue to live out the dreams it spins with ever-increasing energy and economic investment.

Yet for all its successes, medicine in its second era falls short of its own aspirations. There remain a number of great world health problems. The most obvious, and surely the most disturbing, are the still high infant mortality rate, shortened life expectancies, and high sickness rates from infectious diseases and other conditions that mark the health profile of many developing countries. Ominously, as the director of the World Health Organization (WHO) has observed, "we stand on the brink of a global crisis in infectious diseases."[1] Such diseases killed 17 million people in 1995, including 9 million young children. Millions of people die each year from conditions that have been eradicated in the developed countries, and it is the children of the world who suffer the most. At the other end of the life spectrum are the problems of aging societies, heavily burdened by chronic and degenerative disease. The end of life has become a time of growing fear and the occasion of painful moral wrestling about the allocation of resources to the elderly.

Worldwide there is the urgent problem of the increasing number of sick and disabled people, those who in the prescientific era would simply have died but who now live on, alive but not well. China's reported campaign to discourage the birth of the mentally retarded, who because of medical advances can now live into old age, is painfully reminiscent of Nazi Germany's effort to rid itself of the same group over a half century ago; it shows one extreme of the concern. Modern medicine's capacity to save life is greater than its capacity to ensure a healthy, illness-free life for those it has rescued.

The spirit of the era, our own historical setting, is of special importance. There has been ample time now to watch the unfolding of three primary themes, characteristically modern, that mark that spirit. The first is a powerful drive to dominate nature and bring it to heel. Here the legacy of Francis Bacon can be seen. That domination required people to repudiate the passivity and resignation, the fatalism, that had marked the prescientific era. Nature is there to be conquered, and there is no good reason it cannot be conquered. "We cannot," the late Joseph Fletcher wrote in his influential 1954 book *Morals and Medicine*, "submit to physiology and its irrational patterns without abdicating our moral status."[2] Illness and death, it was felt, are correctable biological flaws, destined to yield to scientific ingenuity. Medicine has always nurtured the virtue of hope, but where once it was the only virtue available to cope with unavoidable necessity, hope now became the stuff of

29

change, profit, and unbridled optimism that the human body could be made to reform its errant ways.

The second theme that has shaped the spirit of modern medicine is that of unlimited horizons, of infinite possibilities for ameliorating the human condition. Medicine's future is to be open-ended; it must go as far as it can, and then try to go still further. Who can say what the limits of life extension might really be? Who can say whether it will be possible, through genetic engineering, to improve upon ordinary human nature? Who can say that there might not, someday, be an artificial organ to substitute for every natural organ in a failing human body? The medical enterprise admits to no final and satisfactory resting point. On the contrary, every step of progress opens the way for still more progress, and that progress to still more, indefinitely into the future. Even to admit a possible endpoint is already, in the eyes of many, to compromise the ideal of progress.

The third theme is that of aggressive social expansionism; the social place of medicine has been redefined. First, many have adopted a definition of health that makes it coincide with the drive for happiness and human welfare in general. This is exemplified by the 1947 World Health Organization definition of health: "Health is a state of complete physical, mental, and social well-being and not merely the absence of disease or infirmity." Second, we have expanded the reach of medicine into a wide range of social problems that in earlier times would not have been considered health matters at all. Teenage pregnancy, substance abuse, the psychological stress of ordinary life, and violence are now considered fair game for medical intervention. The domain of medicine expands not only "vertically," to pursue all bodily and emotional goods, but "horizontally," to encompass the relief of an ever-widening range of social ills. Third, we make use of medical skills to increase choice and autonomy, allowing people to improve upon even benign nature, as with cosmetic surgery to enhance appearance; contraception and safe abortion to control childbearing; the use of human growth hormone to help a child achieve greater social competitiveness; and prenatal diagnosis to select the sex of a child.

The second era of medicine, marked by these three themes of modernism in its medical guise, cannot and ought not be continued as a viable enterprise. As the widespread crises of the health care systems of the developed countries should make clear—and none is now exempt from severe stress—open-ended expansionism is increasingly unaffordable, and a source of growing public dissatisfaction. Nature has not been brought to heel, and the very success to date of the effort to gain that kind of mastery has now generated its own set of new problems.

By its tacit implication that in the quest for health lies, perhaps, the secret of the meaning of life, modern medicine has misled people into thinking that the ills of the flesh, and mortality itself, are not to be understood and integrated into a balanced view of life but simply to be fought and resisted. It is as if the medical struggle against illness, aging, and death is itself the source of (or at least *a* source of) human meaning. I refer not only to the almost religious devotion some have to improving their health and their bodies, so that health itself becomes the goal of life, but also to the idea that, in an otherwise meaningless world, the effort to relieve suffering becomes a source of meaning. René Descartes may have unwittingly set medicine on that path in the modern, and popular, mind when he wrote in 1637 that "for the mind depends so much on the temperament and disposition of the bodily organs that, if it is possible to find a means of rendering men wiser and cleverer than they have hitherto been, I believe it is in medicine that it must be sought."[3]

Yet medicine itself is not necessarily at fault for the strain of health-religiosity, or "healthism" as it has sometimes been called, that is part of the contemporary scene. Rather, by hitching itself uncritically to the hubris of modernism (which can in part be traced to Descartes), medicine has created a

31

whole range of incipient problems, but especially the desire for unlimited improvement, which are now being fully expressed. The popular and conventional notion that simply more of the same will overcome these emergent problems can increasingly be seen as a hope with few good foundations. No less implausible is the widespread view that better schemes of health care delivery, different financial incentives, an expanded role for the market, and the elimination of waste can adequately cope with the financial demands made on health care systems. Equity—meaning fair and equal access to decent health care—while achieved in many countries from the 1950s through the 1980s, is beginning to be endangered even where it was at its strongest, in Western Europe, and is disappearing altogether in such countries as Vietnam and China, where it once existed.

Of course health care problems in the developing countries are far more severe than those in the developed countries, and also different in many respects. Many developing nations do not yet face the kinds of high-technology dilemmas that plague the developed countries—a shortage of organ donors, or debates about terminating dialysis treatment, for instance. And although even now, more and more, they face some of them, they may never have the money to afford such moral and social dilemmas to the extent experienced in wealthier countries. Yet even as the developing countries gradually improve their health care systems, they will (and should) have to set goals other than simply catching up with the developed countries. Public health measures and primary care will remain the highest priorities. The problems now being encountered by the developed countries provide, however, important cautionary tales, which if observed carefully can help the developing countries find some alternative pathways, economically and socially more prudent.

In the end, both the developed and the developing countries will have to find new ways out of the second era of medicine and into a third, with different aims and a different spirit—which will encompass a way of life, a set of mores, and a guiding vision. By a "third era" I mean one in which the pre-eminent goal is a medicine and a health care system marked by sustainability, affordability, and equity, one that does not always limit itself to providing traditional care and comfort, but that does tame its aspirations for something infinitely better.

Sustainable Medicine/Sustainable Environment

The environmental movement has given us a concept that can be used fruitfully in a medical context. Environmentalists are now working toward a "sustainable environment." By that they mean an environment that retains its capacity decently to sustain human life over the coming generations, leaving intact the beauty and resources of nature for the needs, satisfaction, and pleasure of future generations. Here and there the terms "steady state" and "sustainable" have already been picked up in medicine. Harold Varmus, the director of the National Institutes of Health (NIH), has said that his organization—the most important government research agency in the world—must learn to live with a "steady-state budget," one that in the future will not automatically increase each year.[4] Discussing the financial crisis in the Medicare program of health care for the elderly—a crisis expected by 2001—Gail R. Wilensky, a former director of the Health Care and Financing Administration, has noted that the central problem is "how to achieve a sustainable level of overall per-person spending on Medicare."[5] The medical economist Rashi Fein follows up that comment by observing that such a development—requiring a cut in resources allocated to elderly health care—cannot be achieved "without substantially impeding the delivery of high-quality health care."[6] True enough. But as environmentalists know all too well, sustainability often forces us to give up things we think important. The same will be true in medicine. I will argue that there is no other choice now available; and that, in any case, we may on balance come out well enough. The health lawyer George Annas was quite perceptive in arguing that over against the mainline models of medicine we now use—notably the economic—environmentalism offers us a different way of casting and articulating our medical problems.[7]

If some astute observers of the medical scene have already begun using the term "sustainable" for parts of the medical and health enterprise, I now want to use it in a much more sweeping way, applying it to the enterprise as a whole. The medical context obviously differs from the environmental. Social, not natural, resources are primarily at stake, and they are more renewable. And while medicine must think of its obligations to future generations, as when it pursues through genetic engineering changes that might be passed on to later generations, the main medical focus will be on the present and the immediate, short-term future. I don't want, then, to claim in my use of the term "sustainable" some tidy parallel with its use in the environmental arena. Instead, I want to suggest that, adapted to the context of medicine and health care, sustainability offers a suggestive and different way of thinking about a wide range of problems facing medicine and health care.

Sustainability is specifically useful in calling attention to the need for a medicine that does not require constant progress or unlimited horizons to be humanly valuable, and which may in fact be harmed by them. Analogously, the environmental movement has tried to alert us to the fundamental tension between the idea of constant economic growth and ever-improved standards of living, and the preservation of a healthy environment. If the growth–some growth–no growth struggle is particularly strong, even virulent, in environmentalism, it would not hurt to see a comparable struggle erupt in medicine. (The environmental movement, I note, now talks of "healthy" and "unhealthy" environments; a useful two-way street may be developing).[8] The notion of sustainability is also fruitful in leading us to think about those basic and minimal conditions necessary for the flourishing of human life. It can no less help us to think about the dangerous price that may be paid for the untrammeled pursuit of an optimal quality of life, a price that in the long run can include a threat to those basic and minimal conditions themselves, a case of the best driving out the good.

Environmentalism has also helpfully tried to recall to our minds the abiding fact that human beings live in, and are themselves a part of, nature. It is a mistake, environmentalists have argued, to think that nature can just be ignored, or over-powered, when our individual and social aspirations push us that way. Medicine itself needs to rethink its relationship to nature, even if (as I will contend in Chapter 4), it cannot follow quite the same course as environmentalism. In short, I am us-ing the concept of sustainability for its suggestive, analogical qualities, not meaning to imply some exact match between medical and environmental issues. I will, in addition, now and then make use of some other helpful environmental concepts in the same way, but not nearly so fully or systematically.

A Working Definition

Let me offer for the purposes of this book a definition of what I mean by "sustainable medicine." (I will embellish it in due course.)

A sustainable medicine will have three characteristics. It will, first, provide the people of a society with a level of medical and public health care sufficient to give them a good chance of making it through the life cycle and of functioning at a decent level of physical and mental competence. It will, second, be a medicine that can be equitably distributed without undue strain, affordable to the society. It must, third, be a medicine that has, with public support, embraced finite and steady-state health goals and has limited aspirations for progress and tech-nological innovation.

A sustainable medicine will not be perfect, nor will it

seek to be. An economically sustainable medicine will of necessity be a medicine of rationing and limits, which, however, are willingly embraced for the sake of sustainability and equity. It will aim for a situation in which a society has reached, and is willing to accept, an adequate but not optimal quality of medicine and level of health, a medicine not addicted to constantly moving forward from adequacy to optimality, much less perfection.

Such a society would recognize that the economic and social costs of even aspiring to an optimal medicine—the satisfaction of *almost every* individual health need, desire, and dream, the pursuit of every research possibility—are dangerously high, a threat to other important societal goods. That society would then be willing to settle for a steady-state medicine, one that was affordable over time, limited and more circumspect in its aspirations, slow in its growth, and willing to forgo possible progress in the name of economic and social stability. Such a society would see a great threat in the expansionary contemporary medicine, a threat not only to its economic life but to a sensible understanding of the place of health in life and of medicine in society.

A sustainable medicine, psychologically, would be one governed by a closed, life-cycle model of individual life—a closed model in the sense that it would not seek indefinite cure of disease or extension of life, either incrementally or decisively, and a life-cycle model in that it would accept different degrees of health and functioning at different stages of life, with the end of life marked by decline and death. Sustainable medicine would accept the continuing, permanent reality of risk, disease, illness, and mortality. It would be a medicine that did not try to overcome those certainties utterly, but shaped a practice and a perspective that had learned how better to adapt to them rather than conquer them. It would foster hope, but circumscribed rather than utopian hope.

A sustainable medicine would, above all, recognize that, in the pattern of health now displayed by the healthiest people in the present developed world, an adequate level of health for now and the future has *already* been reached; it is "good enough" now. An economically sustainable medicine would accept that level as a standard sufficient for a societally acceptable steady-state medicine and a tolerable level of individual health.[9] This point is important in thinking about our obligations to future generations. Surely those generations will have health problems, perhaps many that are different from our own. Those coming generations will be poorly served if we bequeath to them only a medicine addicted to endless improvement. That is the wrong attitude to leave them. It cannot be afforded economically or socially, even if it might be paid for by sacrificing other basic goods. A sustainable medicine, by contrast, would understand that health needs and medical desires must be balanced against other societal priorities—education, jobs, culture, for instance—and that it is foolish to incur economic bankruptcy or excessive stress as the price of deploying their full ambitions and possibilities.

Medicine ought not ad infinitum lure people on to higher and higher expectations or to the generation of ever more insistent needs to keep pace with technological developments. By holding out the possibility of constant improvement—better health, longer lives, less disability—second-era medicine also generates a perverse phenomenon identified years ago by John Knowles: "doing better and feeling worse."[10] A gap of painful consequences has been opened between what people want and hope for from medicine, and what it can actually give them. Whatever it gives them, they want more, yet when they get it they think of themselves as worse, not better off.[11] Such unquenchable wants and never-satisfied hopes are stimulated by the constant hype of new and expected medical breakthroughs, and by constantly raising the threshold of what is thought minimally decent and adequate. A psychologically sustainable medicine would be, at once, less ambitious and more satisfying. It would invite people to live within limits not only of money but of aspiration. Could this kind of medicine generate the type of hope that has marked the second era? No. But it could promise a hope for a good life that was realistic and attainable.

A sustainable medicine is not possible with the spirit that has animated the later phase of the second era. That phase, *our* phase, is breaking the bank and poisoning the spirits of those human beings always caught between the large promise of medicine and the actual life it can bring us. The new goal should, then, be economic and psychological sustainability, out of which should come a more or less steady-state medicine.

What do I mean by a "more or less steady-state medicine"? A "steady-state" medicine is one in which a socially agreed upon proportion of the GNP is devoted to health care, with a set limit (which may be tacit as well as explicit); in which technological changes are slow to come and are rigorously screened for efficacy and affordability; in which changes in the health care system from year to year are relatively slight; in which budgets remain stable (allowed to increase only in proportion to an increase in the GNP or the rate of annual inflation); in which the public for the most part expects only slightly incremental improvement in the level and quality of health care; and in which further scientific gains are not deployed until earlier ones are fully utilized. Almost everyone, in every country, has recognized that health costs cannot increase infinitely and indefinitely. No country can give over its entire GNP to health care. Everyone has, jokingly, always said that. But if that commonsense perception is taken seriously, then an eventual steady-state budget, not always climbing, is the only alternative.

By the phrase "more or less" I mean to suggest that nothing will, or could, stand utterly still; that will be as true of medicine as of automobiles or jet aircraft. But it is the speed of change that is important, and a steady-state medicine will change relatively slowly, allowing time for careful evaluations of its technologies, time to assess various methods of health care delivery, and time to dampen significantly public expectations for continued change in the future. The plateau of a steady-state medicine will probably rise over time, but slowly, undramatically, and in a way relatively undemanding of significant additional social and economic resources.

Getting from Here to There

The way to a sustainable medicine is not exclusively through the play of the market, which even as it promises to control costs, in reality also stimulates the infinite aspirations of second-era medicine, ever seeking new pastures of profit. It is not exclusively through the action of government, whose regulation and budgetary controls can only dampen but not extinguish the drive of medicine to always transcend its earlier condition, let alone the desire of individuals to have their lives improved by medicine. A sustainable medicine is not possible with the economically and psychologically damaging spirit that has animated the later phase, our phase, of the second era.

A sustainable medicine can only come about by a medicine-society dialogue, designed to help medicine rethink its role, its ends, its meaningful goals—that is, by rethinking medicine's inner life and how that life is best understood, and by rethinking its relationship to the society in which it is imbedded. If that can be done—if the underlying substrate of concepts, hopes, aspirations, and serious possibilities can be altered—then the market could have a useful role to play, just as would government. But a government, or a marketplace, that tries to live with the model of medicine given us by the second era will exacerbate rather than help solve the problem.

The implementation of a sustainable medicine lies in two directions. One is the way of prevention, health promotion, and a public health priority. Here the focus will be on reducing the social and environmental problems that are now reckoned to be the most significant source of illness, disease, and premature death. The emphasis will fall on public measures, aimed at improving or sustaining the health of all, seeking a medical common good. The other direction is toward greater personal responsibility for health, laying upon individuals a far stronger obligation (backed by appropriate social and economic incentives) to take care of their health than has been the case with our form of medicine—and, simultaneously, laying upon society a stronger obligation to change those social and economic institutions that generate, or abet, poor health habits. A medicine oriented toward public health on the one hand and greater personal responsibility on the other can be both economically and—with some other changes—psychologically sustainable. Yet, as I will try to show, there are enormous and insufficiently appreciated obstacles in the way of moving in these directions, obstacles both within medicine and outside it (see Chapters 5 and 6).

The most important of these obstacles is technological medicine—that is, the effort to use technology to undo or to minimize the impact of illness and disease. As the medical sociologist David Mechanic has noted, "The irony is that while so much of the challenge in health care is social—to enhance the capacities of individuals to perform desired roles and activities—the thrust of the health care enterprise is substantially technologic and reductionist, treating complex sociomedical problems as if they were amenable to simple technical fixes."[12]

To be sure, there will always be a need for, and certainly a desire for, technological medicine. Not all disease and illness can be coped with by personal efforts or public health programs. The real enemy of a sustainable medicine is the heavy dependence upon and unbridled affection for technology, which has set the character of modern medicine and in great part shaped its research agenda. The dominance of technological medicine has led people to believe that, when all seems lost, medicine can rescue them from their own failings and those of society. The union of technological medicine and the market has immeasurably intensified that belief: the market

sells dreams and hopes as well as things. A sustainable medicine must work to radically reduce this technological dependency, working to show its baneful economic consequences
no less than its dependency-inducing impact on individual behavior and expectations.

I am hardly saying anything wholly new here. Some years
ago, Lewis Thomas spoke of the need to rid ourselves of
halfway technologies—those that save our lives but do not
make us well (his examples were organ transplantation and
kidney dialysis)—and learn better how to find complete cures
or perfect prevention.[13] But Thomas was far too optimistic
about the possibilities for cure, particularly of chronic disease,
and he did not foresee the reemergence of infectious disease.
The cry for better prevention programs and for greater individual responsibility for health is now heard everywhere. But why
has this been said for years to so little avail? A sustainable medicine dependent upon a powerful and salient role for public
health simply cannot be put into practice at present. The values and predispositions of second-era medicine guarantee that
a primary emphasis on prevention, public health, and personal responsibility cannot possibly prevail, even if some minor advances can occur. They will always be seen as add-ons,
always take second place, never be competitive for money or
prestige, never be capable of inflaming the public, and never
be likely to attract the best minds or the best research. That is
what must change.

A serious notion of sustainable medicine must do more
than preach public health and personal responsibility in the
face of the technological domination of medicine. It must be
prepared to divert money and resources away from that form of
medicine and spend them elsewhere. A drastic reallocation of
resources is needed—and to get that effort started, a no less
drastic change in thinking is required. Most of the edifice of
second-era medicine must now be brought down, to be rebuilt
in a sustainable way. The meaning of medicine, and its place
in the lives of individuals and society, must be changed. Medi-

cine must be transformed from the inside so that when money is reallocated from the outside the change will seem sensible, not offensive—as it surely would at present.

My aim is to look at the moral and social foundations of modern medicine and the way it understands the world, and then to find those points of intellectual and scientific leverage necessary to bring about change, a change that will take us into the third era. We will have to open up once again the ancient Greek struggle between *hygeia*, the belief that the body, if well and prudently tended, can take care of and cure itself, and *aesculapius*, the contrasting belief that only a medical intervention can set the body straight. Over forty years ago, René Dubos's great book *Mirage of Health*, which I have already mentioned, called our attention to this struggle, pointing out how it enacted itself throughout the history of medicine but how, in our time, *aesculapius* has triumphed.[14] The idea of *hygeia* needs to be brought to life again, not simply because it has merit in its own right but also because the effort to create a greater sense of personal responsibility for health needs the motivation of likely personal success no less than the motivation of economic necessity.

We have, as a modern people, come to believe that only technological medicine can save us, can overcome the failings of a body thought incomplete, fatally flawed, and otherwise biologically doomed. A peculiar feature of our individualistic Western society, bent on all forms of personal liberation, is that we have been willing to put our medical fate in the hands of others, those who manage the technological fixes, rather than take unto ourselves the healing of the self. There are signs that this is beginning to change, but such change needs a great deal of stimulation to give it significant momentum.

If, at one end of the spectrum, the self and society must increasingly look to themselves to maintain health, in the collective provision of health care there must be still another, and contrasting, virtue: that of human solidarity in the face of their common fate of sickness and death. The idea of solidarity has been the sustaining moral and political note of European health care systems, guaranteeing to all citizens equal and decent access to health care. That note needs a fresh breath of vitality. It has never gained real footing in the United States — where the language of rights, and specifically of a "right" to health care, is thought preferable — or in the developing countries. It is now also under severe stress in those European countries that are its home, where it is threatened by a fraying of the welfare state and by the consequent inroads of medical privatization and the pull of the market. For the developing countries, however, and even for those developed countries tempted to give it up, solidarity still remains the best — and, indeed, *only* plausible — foundation for a potent public health system and, beyond that, for the common provision of medical care.

Yet to give the combination of self-reliance and solidarity sufficient bite to change the way medicine is practiced and health care delivered, and to create from it a sustainable medicine, requires foundational work. The medicine of the second historical era has behind it a distinctive stance toward progress, toward technological innovation, toward nature, and toward the self, society, and suffering. Unless that stance can be changed, little else is likely to be altered. In that stance medicine has defined itself in relationship to the most basic human needs and the place of human life in nature. Modern medicine rests, that is, on a philosophy of both external nature and human nature. That philosophy generates the emotional trajectory of modern medicine, full of self-stimulated optimism and often gross hubris. It no less importantly frames the way medicine looks at the possibilities of nature and the self, the latter situated in a position of assumed dominance and unlimited manipulative capacities. Technology gives us the power to dominate nature, and when technology goes awry, it is technology that, many believe, can also supply the antidote. Technological ideology is, in that sense, a self-referential and closed world: what it can do it can undo, and what it can make it can remake, and what it can envision it can reenvision. It needs only itself to manage itself.

Modern medicine rests on a view of the self that perfectly mirrors, and makes zealous use of, the ideology of technology. The self of modern medicine is no less open in its possibilities than the medicine it uses to realize them: it is a protean self, the creation of its own capacities to make of human beings what they would like to be. Most of all, they would like to be free of the constraints of nature, which gives them too much suffering, too much illness, too early a death, too many children, too much genetic determinism, and too precarious a hold on a life of their own choosing. If medicine is to change, then its view of the self must be changed as well.

Yet to change the way medicine thinks of the self will make it into still another realm, that of medicine in its relationship to society. There is no isolated self. All of us are imbedded in particular cultures and societies, shaped and tutored by them. The self that we fashion will in great part be fashioned for us by that context. The self of modern medicine is no less a product of a culture, one which has seen the binding of liberal ideas of individuals and their relationship to society spliced with the scientific and technological possibilities of medicine. They have needed and fed on each other. The classical model of modern scientific medicine focuses on the welfare of the individual (which is part of the reason it has trouble encompassing a public health model), but it should be evident by now that medicine helps shape the larger society in which that individual exists. Medicine's capacity to change that society will have as much impact on what becomes of individuals as will medicine's focus on the individual per se. It may even have more.

The great mediating force here, working back and forth between the self and society, is technology. It puts before our eyes new medical and human possibilities, giving us more choice, more opportunities for good health, and more ways of playing with our human nature. How a technological medicine—existing in a technological society and working with a protean modern self that looks to technology for transforming possibilities—should be understood and if possible reshaped must be part of any effort to make sense of the future goals of a sustainable medicine. The place to start an examination of technological medicine is with the idea of progress.

CHAPTER TWO

Arguing with Success: Progress and the Medical Dream

It is said that you can't argue with success. But you can and I will. For all its triumphs, medicine's pursuit of unlimited progress has reached that point at which its old success story has begun to look shopworn but a new one has yet to be born.* Nor will the new story easily come to birth. The continuing power of medicine to capture our imagination, to spoonfeed us a steady dose of mostly small but sometimes striking successes and larger promissory notes of greater triumphs still

---

*When I speak of "medicine," I do not mean to imply that everyone in medicine has such values. I am trying, instead, to characterize the historical dynamism and language of modern scientific medicine: its most common, mainline values. Though these remain dominant, they are by no means the only tradition of values. On the contrary, over against the medicine I am critical of is the important tradition stressing the patient as person, the power of the body to heal itself, the need for caring and compassion. A sustainable medicine will need a strong underpinning of those medical values.

to come, is formidable. The old story continues to look viable, sustained by the still-vivid memory of its past achievements, whose fruits greet us daily at the door of the doctor's office, the clinic, and the hospital: the impressive diagnostic technique, the helpful drug, the life-saving organ transplant. But there is even more: Vice President Al Gore has written in the journal *Science* of the "virtuous circle of progress and prosperity," thus harnessing progress to economic well-being, a cause hardly less dear than that of health.[1] Health, progress, and prosperity are a sweet mix.

Those who would joust with such formidable forces face a difficult struggle. The argument of this chapter, nonetheless, is that a sustainable medicine demands a far-ranging critique of the idea of straight-line, unlimited progress. That idea lies at the heart of modern medicine, a fount of hope, a prod to ambition, and a source of considerable economic benefits. Nothing less than some conception of an alternative, sustainable notion of progress must be articulated and pursued. My aim is to pursue four questions: How might the modern medical dream, with its roots in the idea of progress, best be characterized? What are the emergent biological obstacles to unlimited progress? What have been the harmful consequences of an unwillingness to take those obstacles seriously? What might an alternative, sustainable idea of progress look like? In the next chapter I will look at the related notion of innovative technology, but it is the idea of progress that is the source of just about everything else, and it is there that one ought to begin.

Why should anyone want to challenge the idea of unlimited medical progress? Because modern medicine, including its successes as well as its failures, is well on the way to becoming economically insupportable and socially hazardous. This may seem a harsh and pessimistic assessment, particularly in light of the gains in health that modern biological and technological knowledge have given us. Yet such an assessment makes sense only *because* of the great advances of medicine, its undoubted progress, which have taken us to levels undreamed of by earlier generations. Precisely because it has come so far, medicine has assumed that the future will go as well as the past—and therein lies the error. Medicine has failed to consolidate and well exploit the gains already made and, what is no less important, has assumed it can extrapolate comparable progress into the future.

The evidence is now suggesting, however, that it is a fundamental mistake to generalize from the success of the past to assume like gains in the future. As George Washington once noted, It "would be . . . unreasonable to suppose that because a man has rolled a snowball till it acquired the size of a horse that he might do so till it was as large as a house."[2] Success there will surely be, and medical progress as well. But (a) the future is unlikely to hold great gains such as there were in the past—that is, medical gains that have a decisive *population* health benefit; (b) future advances will be proportionately far more expensive to find and to implement than those of the past; and (c) future advances will be considerably more likely to be ambiguous, perhaps even contradictory, in their human benefits.

An analogy comes to mind. Medical progress is not inherently different from the exploration of outer space. No matter how far one goes, there is always farther one can go. The burden of going farther out into space, like that of continuing medical progress on top of past progress, is accumulating costs: it costs nothing to jump a foot off the ground, considerably more to put humans in orbit around the earth, still more to mount a moon exploration project, and exponentially more to send human beings beyond the moon to far more distant planets.

Understood in this vein, it is not the initiation or early stages of medical progress that pose the problem, but its indefinite continuation. If we had not made so much medical progress in the past, had not come so far, had not been so successful, we would not now be facing the escalating costs, human and economic, of trying to keep pace with the past. Just because of those costs we need to reconsider the original dream, to see where it fails to serve us any longer and where, in fact, hanging on to it too long becomes even harmful.

As Daniel Sarewitz has noted, no myth is so powerful as that of the "infinite benefit" of research, the belief that "the more we spend on research the better our quality of life will be."[3] The close analogue here is the no less hardy myth that the more medical progress we have, the better off we will be, and that medical progress always brings more benefits than problems, more gains than losses. These myths may have some foundation in reality, but they are far from proven even with respect to past gains, and even less well demonstrated with respect to the supposed future benefits of medical progress. It may be that no proof in a strict sense is required. Perhaps it is enough that progress is an attractive, hopeful dream, with sufficient credibility to keep us moving. Even so, we need to look carefully at it. Even as we do so, we should keep in mind an incisive observation of the great sociologist Max Weber some eighty years ago in his lecture "Science as a Vocation." It is of the essence of scientific achievement, he wrote, that "it *asks* to be surpassed and out dated."[4] That is surely as true of medical science, which wants always to know more, and cure better, than it did in the past. Hence, even though I will here stress the problems with medicine's dream of progress, the fact of continued suffering and death helps to keep it alive.

Medicine's Dream of Progress

What is the modern medical dream of progress? It is less easy to answer that question than one might guess, but René Descartes's optimistic speculation in 1637 is as pertinent today as when he wrote it, perhaps even more so: "I am sure that there is no one . . . who does not confess that all that men know is almost nothing in comparison with what remains to be known; and that we could be free of an infinitude of mal-

adies both of body and mind, and even also possibly of the in-
firmities of age, if we had sufficient knowledge of their causes,
and of all the remedies with which nature has provided us."[5]
Descartes's optimism is easily matched by a contemporary
physician, Michael Fossel: "We will be able to prevent, even
reverse, aging within two decades. At the same time, and as
part of the same progress, we will also cure most of the diseases
that now frighten and destroy us."[6]

Despite a persistent utopian strain over the centuries,
there is nowhere written some single charter of progress for
the modern medical enterprise, agreed upon by researchers,
clinicians, and the general public. There have been comparatively few efforts to formally articulate specific goals for
medicine. It has been sufficient simply to say, as did a former
director of the National Institutes of Health, that medicine
seeks "to maintain health, relieve human suffering, and prevent death from disease."[7]

But what exactly do those goals *mean?* Here the picture
becomes hazy and the actual working goals have emerged
more from the practice of medicine than from theoretical efforts to define medical purposes. We can seek through medical
progress:

- to understand the biological and other causes of disease

- to reduce mortality rates and thereby extend life
  expectancy in general and the lives of individuals in particular

- to achieve greater equality of death and sickness outcomes among different groups of people

- to reduce or eliminate the causes of disease and illness

- to ameliorate the effects of illness and disability through
  rehabilitation and palliation

- to relieve the pain and suffering of accidents and illness

- to develop greater diagnostic capacities for present disease

- to predict the probabilities of future disease

If those are the major goals of medical progress, scientific research and technological innovation are commonly assumed to be the principal means of accomplishing them. Basic research seeks to understand the root causes of disease, illness, and disability, while medical technology provides the practical means for coping with them. That technology includes medical stratagems (therapeutic, palliative, rehabilitative, pharmaceutical, for instance); diagnostic devices (machines and screening instruments); and information systems (computers, most notably). Progress, both in research and in technological applications, can be either great and dramatic (the discovery of a polio vaccine), or gradual and incremental (treatments for childhood cancers). What seems most striking about the medical dreams in the scientific literature (as distinguished from science fiction) is not the projection of some generally improved human state or human nature. Science's dreams for medicine appear instead as a set of incremental improvements, focused on this or that discrete condition or malady one by one; the advances do not sum as a unified goal for the medical enterprise.

This dream of progress has varied aims, which we might call traditional and utopian. The traditional aim is to find cures for, or to ameliorate, physical and psychological conditions that cause death, pain, suffering, and the loss of characteristic human functioning. "Normal" good health is the goal. The utopian dream is to use medical knowledge to satisfy the desire to transcend physical and psychological problems that stand in the way of realizing human goals and aspirations other than that of improved health—a better memory, or dramatically longer lives, or less violence, or greater intelligence, for instance. Optimal health is the aim here, health that is not only sufficient for the good functioning of the organism but that gives an added boost to other human goals.

Whether the dream is stated in a traditional or a utopian way, we must understand that it is, in modern hands, open-ended and inherently expansionist. To use the concepts of the historian of science Gerald Holton, it aims for both omni-science (a unified theory of the causes of disease) and omnipo-tence (the overpowering of disease).[8] The dream of medical progress does not have any logical or obvious endpoint or any intrinsic constraints. Nor is it at all clear just what would count as a full realization of the dream. The eradication of all suffering? The cure of every disease? An endless old age? Im-mortality? When asked about the goals of the labor move-ment, the nineteenth-century union leader Samuel Gompers is reputed to have said, "More!" If modern medicine had a sin-gle collective voice it would probably say something like that: there is no ultimate end point, just *more* cure, *more* relief or suffering, *more* success in holding off death. In *The Idea of Progress*, the historian J. B. Bury wrote that "you have not got the idea of progress until you go on to conceive that it is des-tined to advance indefinitely in the future."[9]

Precisely because modern medicine's unspoken goal is simply *more*, there are no limits to what can be hoped for and sought. The very absence of any more clearly and precisely ar-ticulated goals fuels the entire enterprise. In modern medi-cine's dream of progress, there are no set boundaries to what societies and individuals can desire, nor to what may be done to satisfy those desires. This is a fine example of what Thomas Sowell has called an "unconstrained vision."[10]

The resolute and welcomed absence of any final goal is it-self a great attraction; it means that there is nothing against which to measure desire, much less to curb it, and nothing to stand in the way of medicine inventing whatever goals it might want from one historical era to another—or of society inventing its own goals for medicine. Precisely this was the form of progress espoused by the historian E. H. Carr, which he took to be essential to the survival of human society. We could, he argued, look forward to improvements "subject to no limits that we can envisage, towards goals that can only be defined as we advance towards them."[11] This is a perfect charter statement for the dream of medical progress, echoed as well by J. B. Bury when he noted that in "achieving its ascendancy and unfolding its meaning, the Idea of Progress had to overcome a psychological obstacle which may be described as *the illusion of finality.*"[12] No one in medicine has used quite such decisive language, but its content is implicit in medicine's quest.

The Dynamics of Progress

To be fully grasped, the medical dream of progress needs to be set within the context of the historical idea of progress as it has developed in the West. A way into that larger domain of progress is nicely offered by comparing two contemporary commentators on the idea of progress, representing different and opposed perspectives: the late sociologist Robert Nisbet and the late cultural historian Christopher Lasch.

Nisbet begins his comprehensive and lucid *History of the Idea of Progress* by trying to show, against the views of an older generation of historians, that the idea of progress can be traced back to Greek and Roman thought. It was by no means the entire invention of the Enlightenment thinkers of the eighteenth century, although they gave it the form and direction most influential thereafter. Nisbet defines the idea of progress as the conviction that "*mankind has advanced in the past—from some aboriginal condition of primitiveness, barbarism, or even nullity—is now advancing, and will continue to advance through the foreseeable future* [italics in original]."[13] He cites the thought of J. B. Bury that the idea of progress encompasses both a perspective on the past, which is one of synthesizing through time earlier human achievements, and a prophecy about the future, which sees more inevitably to come. To this Nisbet adds that "the idea must not be thought the companion of mere caprice or accident; it must be thought a part of the very scheme of things in universe and society. Advance from the inferior to the superior must seem as real and certain as anything in the laws of nature."[14]

Nisbet then asks what this advance from inferior to superior means. His answer is that it in part includes a slow, gradual, and cumulative increase in *knowledge*. The very nature of knowledge "is to advance, to improve, to become more perfect."[15] The other part of the idea of progress is that of an *improvement in the human condition*, most notably moral and spiritual advancement; freedom "from the torments of nature and society"; and "serenity or tranquillity." Despite setbacks— from the corruptions of totalitarian political schemes or the unintended and unforeseen consequences of some forms of progress (environmental pollution caused by automobiles, or population pressures generated by the much-desired reduction in infant mortality, for example)—Nisbet wrote: "I remain convinced that this idea has done more good over a twenty-five-hundred-year period . . . than any other single idea in Western history."[16] The idea of progress, he held, is a "dogma" and a "faith," not itself scientific, but primarily benign and salubrious in its history and consequences.

Nisbet concluded his history by noting many recent challenges to the idea of progress. They include the negative reactions that surfaced widely during the early part of the twentieth century—among the intellectuals Søren Kierkegaard, Max Weber, Georges Sorel, the Adams brothers in America, Oswald Spengler, and the writers T. S. Eliot, James Joyce, Ezra Pound, and William Butler Yeats. He did not note, but well could have, the burst of an antitechnology spirit—the "greening" of America—that was a feature of the 1960s and 1970s, notably expressed in the writings of Theodore Roszak, Charles Reich, and the final works of Lewis Mumford. More recently, a spate of authors have suggested that progress itself, good or bad, may be coming to an end. The molecular biologist Gunther Stent has argued that "progress really *is* nearing its end in our time. . . . My principal reason for this conclusion was that progress embodies several internal contradictions—psychological, material, and epistemological—which render it self-limiting."[17] The Czech writer Ivan Klíma sees the phenomenon as more generally an end to our era: "An age that rated so highly virtues such as rapid development, competitiveness, change, progress, innovation, and modernity, often at the expense of other values, is over."[18]

But prophecies of the death of the idea of progress are premature; perhaps they always will be. Christopher Lasch, who shared neither Nisbet's enthusiasm nor Stent and Klíma's radical judgment, nonetheless offered a dark assessment. His 1991 book, *The True and Only Heaven: Progress and Its Critics*, published a decade later than Nisbet's, brought together in a comprehensive way his thinking about progress. For Lasch, it made no sense to entertain a nostalgic view of the past as a way of overcoming the "persistence of a belief in progress in a century full of calamities."[19] Those calamities did not, and will not, deter the pursuit of more progress any more than invoking a more benign past will. The challenge instead is to find a source of hope that does not depend upon satisfying insatiable wants. "Progressive optimism," Lasch wrote, "rests, at bottom, on a denial of the natural limits of human power and freedom, and it cannot survive too long in a world in which an awareness of those limits has become inescapable."[20] Once we have become aware of these limits, we need to "recover a more vigorous form of hope, which trusts life without denying its tragic character or attempting to explain away tragedy as a 'cultural lag.'"[21]

I wish I could share Lasch's optimism about the power of an awareness of limits. But there are many tried-and-true ways of evading a message of limits: by accusing the messengers of pathological pessimism, or Ludditism, or simply by asking for more time—an indefinite period of time—to work through the problems that progress can generate. Lasch himself noted the way in which earlier defenders of progress eventually gave up faith in some kind of final heaven on earth and adopted a more modest but still exceedingly potent alternative: the postulation of an indefinite expansion of desire accompanied by a corresponding rise in, and democratically distributed standard of, comfort.[22] Lasch was not happy with this alternative. He held to the very end his ideal of a recovery of hope grounded in acceptance of tragedy. Only that way of thinking, he felt, could possibly cope with the nine lives of an idea of progress that could not easily be put aside for something better, or falsified as untrustworthy.

The idea of medical progress has had an easier time of it than other forms of scientific progress. It has not had to live down nuclear weapons, as physics has had to do; and if the eugenics movements of the late nineteenth and early twentieth centuries scarred the reputation of the biological sciences, more recent genetic medicine has worked hard, and with great success, to overcome that bad memory by putting something scientifically and morally better in its place. Medical progress, moreover, has produced such palpably important gains in human health during the twentieth century that it has only now and then been subject to the fundamental criticism and disillusionment that progress in general had to put up with in the early decades of this century.

Medical progress has had the further advantage of working to rid human life of evils acknowledged by all. If many visions of progress have been, as Lasch noted, of a growth of affluence and a general improvement in the conditions of human life, countervoices—sometimes religious, sometimes aesthetic—have always at least expressed doubt that human beings would actually be better off with the kind of progress sought by the Enlightenment, particularly the kind of affluence espoused by Adam Smith and the followers of a market ideology. Medical progress, by contrast, has had no serious critics; few have questioned the notion that improved health is a human good. Nisbet sees progress in general as expanding freedom, on the one hand, and increasing human power, on the other. The attraction of medical progress is that it does both in spades. It has given people much greater freedom in the face of biological restrictions, and more choice in a world bent on expanded choice. It has no less achieved great power over the forces of nature, which grind us down, sicken us, and ultimately kill us.

Modern medicine helps to create, even as it feeds on, cultural values that give it a high place. Possibly the most potent value might be called the moral imperative of progress: if the human condition can be improved, then there is a moral obligation to seek that improvement. At the same time, the human benefit represented by the ideal of good health and the cure of disease is the kind of transcendent value that will be accorded a relatively high place in any society. No human institution has a higher social status in modernized, free societies than medicine. It controls life and death, matters that no society can ignore and with which every person must cope. At the same time, medical advances and organized health care delivery provide excitement, jobs, and a strong sense of doing good—that is, they satisfy many other desires of society.

It is hardly an accident that those societies most committed to the value of democratic individualism—to the satisfaction of individual preferences without moral judgment of the value of those preferences—spend the most money on medicine and health care and, in particular, look to medicine to remove biological obstacles to the satisfaction of private desires. In the use of medicine to control procreation, to manage mood and affect, and to rescue people from the folly of their personal choices and hazardous lifestyles, modern medicine allows individualism a range of expression that would otherwise be inconceivable. The affluent can turn to medicine for lifestyle therapy, and the poor (if they can afford it) for amelioration of the effects of their poverty.

Though often attacked by outside critics and frequently deplored even by those within the field, the fragmenting, reductionistic, mechanistic model that dominates modern scientific medicine is, in fact, one of its attractions. By presupposing a malleable, manipulable, and mechanistic model of human biology, it draws upon the familiar and highly tractable image of the machine, which can be made to serve—with precision—human need. It is a familiar model in technological societies, understandable and accessible, making progress perspicuous to all, even if the technical details may be obscure. The reductionism of modern medicine serves useful ends as well, allowing us to simplify, disaggregate, and segregate our problems—that is, to cut them down to size and bring them within our grasp. For many medical conditions, moreover, the model works exceedingly well—for the eradication of lethal bacteria, for instance, or for coping with kidney failure.

Yet modern medicine could not possibly have achieved its present social power had not business discovered that there are potentially enormous profits and a good living to be made through medicine and health care. The Enlightenment's joining of scientific and material progress finds a present exemplar in modern commercial medicine. Much of business, of course, builds upon the satisfaction of basic human needs and desires, and it has long been taken for granted that business will not only satisfy desire but also stimulate it. If labor wants "more," so does management and so do stockholders. In the instance of medicine, business finds an ideal situation: powerful and potentially unlimited demand combined with constant scientific progress and technological innovation. Medicine provides jobs and profit, an attractive combination in commercial societies. The final, and crowning, touch is offered by the widespread belief that progress is a moral imperative, not simply a discretionary matter.[23]

Ought medicine to seek, through basic and applied research, further knowledge in order to improve human health? Absolutely. Not only would it be foolish to predict that research could not gain much greater knowledge than it has at present, but also there is no practical way to stop the quest for such knowledge, even if a radical scarcity of money could slow and cripple it.

The question I am raising, however, is not whether further knowledge and medical progress are human goods—they are—but whether we can devise an understanding of progress that contributes to a sustainable, not an economically and often socially reckless, medicine. As presently pursued, and as constantly watered by the aspirations of the modern self and its nurturing society, the reigning idea of medical progress is the single most important barrier to sustainability. I want to see if I can offer a notion of progress that might take its place. My point of departure will be the biological obstacles that progress must now face. I will consider why taking them more seriously would serve well as the beginning of—and a powerful motive to seek—a new common sense about the future of medical progress.

The Struggle Against Biology and Human Nature

The first and most conventional target of modern medical aspiration is the most obvious fact of human biology: bodily decline followed by death. We human beings sicken, age, wither, and die. If we are fortunate, we will make it through a reasonably long life; if not, we will suffer a premature death. Medicine has set its face against death, and hardly less against those injuries, sicknesses, and disease that bring pain, suffering, and disability. To this list must be added one additional general item: medicine has of late also turned its face, on request, against those human conditions that bespeak not illness or bodily failures but the absence of some perceived good that some human beings want: a better appearance (cosmetic surgery), an enhanced sense of well-being (one use of Prozac), or greater height (human growth hormone). When we speak of medical progress, then, we ordinarily mean the possibility of eliminating, or dominating, or ameliorating, some feature of the human body or mind we find below par (however we may define that) or that is open to improvement.

Now, in the nature of the case, it is impossible to rationally imagine a human body that will not be subject to injury, illness, or disease. I say "rationally imagine" to emphasize what is scientifically reasonable to expect in, say, the next century or so. Like it or not, human beings will remain within the realm of organic life, subject to decay, entropy, and the ultimate undoing that is death. If this is so, then my question is this: how much more progress is it *reasonable* to think possible, or to expect under the most prudent forecasts, in medicine's struggle against the finiteness of organic human nature?

In asking this question, my working assumption is this: on many important fronts medicine is now running up against some formidable biological obstacles, of a kind certain to greatly, and increasingly, complicate future progress. Advances made in one domain, moreover, are often offset by regressions or by new problems in other domains.

My question about reasonable possibility must at once be qualified, broken into two parts. The first is this: what are the *theoretical* limits of medical progress in overcoming human biology? There is a short answer to that question, as befits our ignorance: who knows? If the history of science in general, and medicine in particular, has shown us anything, it is that just about nothing is impossible, including the unimaginable. But if a sustainable medicine is our concern, what matters is the second part of the question: what kind of progress and innovation is reasonably likely and feasible *given what we presently know and seem likely to know in the near future of the next few decades?* By that standard of judgment, we should focus our attention on (a) the theoretical building blocks that are already in place or near at hand to make the foreseeable progress a feasible, not wildly speculative, possibility; (b) the research work that is going on in a way and at a pace likely to enhance the possibility that the progress will indeed take place; and (c) those features of the progress that would make realistically possible a less expensive, more sustainable medicine.

Let me now try to apply this standard. I want to ask what kind of progress it is reasonable to expect in the context of five basic categories: the struggles against death, against infectious disease, against chronic illness and disability, against the increased morbidity that has historically accompanied aging, and against the genetic causes of disease.

1. Wrestling with Death. Death has come to be the principal enemy of modern medical progress. Hardly any statistic is more favorably cited in medicine than the striking increase in human longevity, particularly over the past century. Life expectancy in the developed countries of the world has gone from the mid-forties to the mid- to late seventies; in the developing countries, there have also been remarkable improvements. Even sub-Saharan Africa, with the world's worst health, has seen a ten-year increase in life expectancy since 1950, from the low forties to the mid-fifties.[24] In addition to the general, global increase in longevity—primarily the result of lower infant and child mortality rates—there has been a sharp increase in the number and proportion of those over age eighty and even over one hundred. And if statistically not important for overall longevity, the fact that some people now live to be 105 or 110 or even, in one striking case, over 120, is still testimony to possibilities that would have seemed out of the question only a few decades ago.

There are two important scientific issues here. One of them bears on the likely limits, if any, of average human life expectancy. Does the fact that some groups (Japanese women, for example) live *on average* into their early eighties—at the far tail of the life-expectancy bell curve—indicate that they are near or have reached the upper limit of the *average life expectancy* that might eventually be possible for everyone? The

61

other issue is whether the fact that some individuals now live as long as 110 or 120 years indicates that they have reached the outer ring of *individual longevity*, close to or at that limit?

There is no scientific consensus on either issue. The theory of a compression of mortality—that average life expectancy will increasingly cluster at a fixed age—has not been borne out by the evidence.[25] Average life expectancy continues to increase, though gradually and not dramatically.[26] At the same time, the theory that eighty-five will probably mark the upper limit of average life expectancy does not find consistent scientific support either. The upward creep of average life expectancy offers no suggestion that it must necessarily reach some final point. Nor is the significance of the fact that more and more individuals are living well beyond one hundred years wholly clear either. It surely demonstrates that the tail of the life expectancy curve is longer than anyone would have guessed possible in the past, just as it demonstrates the foolhardiness of predicting where the outer limit might finally be—if there is to be some final outer limit at all. It seems, in short, safest to say that we do not yet know what average life expectancy could become in the future, or how long some particularly fortunate (if that is the right term) individuals might live. There is no way of telling whether we are near to, or far from, either of those limits.

What does seem clear (I will develop the point further in the next chapter) is that, if science has yet to discern the biological limits of human life, medicine has not discerned how it can go much beyond its present knowledge and technology to directly and deliberately help reach those limits.[27] Save for some as yet unknown possibilities for genetic manipulation, there is little chance that medical advances as such do, or will, contribute *greatly* to a longer life, either for groups or individuals. Instead, general improvement in living standards and improved health behavior will more likely make the greatest difference. There remains in particular little substance to the prediction that we will move "Forward to Methuselah," the title of an essay in *The Economist* touting soon-to-be medical knowledge that might stop aging and lead to 300-year life spans.[28]

Not even the most radical forecasts predict for the twenty-first century an increase in life expectancy of the magnitude—about thirty years—that marked the twentieth century; this is in great part because it was the striking reduction in infant mortality rates that accounted for the increase. Infant mortality is not expected to go much lower. At the same time, it should be noted that death rates for all age groups are continuing to decline in developed countries, a trend discernible in many developing countries as well. But this is much more likely caused by general improvements in education and income and other background conditions than by specifically medical contributions—which, though not absent, of course, are less decisive in their impact.

If there are formidable difficulties now in trying to deliberately extend by medical means average life expectancy at the end of life, comparable obstacles appear at the beginning of life. As I pointed out in the preceding paragraph, a great portion of the twentieth century's increase in life expectancy was the result of decreased infant mortality. In the developed countries infant mortality is now low, under 10 per 1,000 live births, and the annual gains in general are now slight. The problems encountered with low-birthweight and premature babies illustrate the appearance of still another biological barrier to progress. Prematurely born babies, of twenty-three to twenty-four weeks' gestation and weighing as little as 450 to 500 grams, can now sometimes be saved, occasionally with good health prospects but usually not. Whether to work aggressively to save such babies is a well-known and difficult moral dilemma.

It seems generally agreed, however, that the art and science of neonatal medicine will not in the foreseeable future do much better, still less do so at a generally affordable cost. The immature lung development of infants at that stage of life has proved to be a profound barrier to viability; it can be chemically overcome to some degree, but not decisively. Short of a highly expensive and as yet undeveloped artificial placenta, the only progress possible in the near term will be minute, and expensive, incremental gains.[29]

Medical progress has, in short, reached some formidable obstacles in the significant deliberate extension of longevity or life span, at both the beginning and end of life.

2. *Infectious Disease.* Until the early twentieth century, most deaths were caused by infectious disease — whether by large-scale plagues and outbreaks of smallpox, yellow fever, typhoid, typhus, influenza, or cholera, or by the more mundane bacterial or viral illnesses of tuberculosis, pneumonia, or dysentery. Infectious disease took a particularly deadly toll among the young, contributing to their high mortality rate, but as a walk through any old cemetery will reveal, it struck people down at all ages. By the middle of the twentieth century, however, the war against infection seemed at an end, at least in the developed countries; this was widely hailed as a triumph of the vaccines that had begun to appear by the end of the nineteenth century, and of the antibiotic and antimicrobial drugs that came out of the 1940s and 1950s. Only in the cases of malaria and some tropical diseases did the conquest appear less than complete, but even with them progress was slowly being made.

Yet a disturbing surprise was in store for a medicine that had all too confidently declared the demise of infectious disease. By the 1980s the emergence of HIV disease was the most striking sign that all was not well after all. Nature showed that it was still capable of throwing up an infectious viral disease of staggering dimensions, seemingly fatal to all who contracted it and so far resistant either to medical prevention by inoculation or to a decisive medical cure. At best, HIV disease might today be described as a formerly quick-acting fatal infectious disease that is gradually being turned into a more slowly lethal chronic disease.

Nor was HIV the only surprise nature had in store for medicine. Deaths from infectious disease are on the increase in the United States.[30] And malaria has staged a comeback in many parts of the world, as have tuberculosis and pneumococcal infections.[31] Bacterial strains have been regularly appearing that are resistant to the postwar antibiotics, even to those later-generation antibiotics developed to cope with the resistance. In the case of a few widely infectious conditions, once the easy target of numerous antibiotics, only one or two effective treatments now exist, and there is considerable worry about how long they will last.

A widely praised 1995 book by Laurie Garrett, *The Coming Plague*, detailed these developments: "microbes," she observed, "[possess] multitudinous ways to outwit any given antibiotic"; and those ways have become a regular feature of medical and scientific reporting.[32] When René Dubos noted in *Mirage of Health*—at just that moment when infectious disease seemed ready to disappear—that nature would constantly generate new pathogens, it seemed a gratuitously pessimistic assessment. But he was absolutely right.[33] Whatever the future of the struggle against infectious diseases, one thing is certain: they are likely never to be fully conquered. The only matter in doubt is how frequently new bacterial and viral strains will appear, and with what virulence. As the biologist Paul W. Ewald has noted, it is a "mistake to interpret disease as a temporary state of imbalance in an otherwise balanced nature."[34] The same point has been richly developed by another biologist, Marc Lappé, when he writes that the "evolutionary message is that we remain at risk for disease in spite of our medical advances. The interconnectedness of all living things on earth . . . is the basis of our continuing peril."[35]

3. *Chronic Disease.* Even though infectious disease is staging a comeback, the leading killers are now the chronic and degenerative diseases characteristic of aging societies. Heart disease, cancer, stroke, and diabetes are the leading causes of death

among the old (and 75 percent of people in developed countries live more than sixty-five years), and take the lives, as well, of many who are still young. For a time, the kind of euphoria that marked the seeming victory over infectious disease was expectantly carried into the domain of chronic diseases, with their conquest predicted as the next likely and logical outcome of medical research.

That conquest has not happened, and there is good reason to doubt that it ever will: the human body inexorably ages and will die of *some* disease or other. From a global perspective, hardly anything is more striking than what has been called the "epidemiological transition" in the developing countries, as the shift from infectious disease to chronic and degenerative disease, once a mark of more affluent nations, now comes to all nations, rich and poor.[36] The death rate from cardiovascular disease has declined significantly for all age groups, and that is a trend often rightly celebrated. Yet if people do not die so frequently from heart disease, its prevalence and morbidity remain high, as does the cost of care for those who develop it.[37] The people being saved from heart disease are usually not people cured of it; they are people allowed now to survive but whose lives will be marked by chronic heart disease.

Cancer presents no less complex a picture. Some of the leukemias and a number of other forms of cancer now have a high cure rate, and in general young people have a much better chance of being cured than was earlier the case. The survival time of those with diagnosed cancer has improved as well. But the more general truth is that the overall death rate from cancer has not decreased in any *significant* way (though it *is* decreasing), especially among the elderly, and there is no sign that the prevalence of cancer is likely to decline in the foreseeable future.[38] Diabetes still kills thousands each year even though its prevalence has apparently stabilized. The incidence of Alzheimer's disease, a particular scourge among the old, has continued to increase with the aging of the population, particularly among the growing numbers of those over eighty-five (of whom 50 percent are now suspected of having some form of dementia).

There are no longer responsible observers or researchers who predict an early end to the chronic and degenerative diseases. If they could once be found, during the 1960s and 1970s in particular, their ranks are now depleted. There is no scientific basis for easy optimism. The causes of cancer, and possible cures, remain almost as elusive today as they were two or three decades ago. More is known, to be sure, particularly at the genetic level, but that knowledge has yet to be translated into decisively effective treatments. Even if an end to the scourge of smoking—the main cause of the leading form of cancer, lung cancer—was at hand, other forms of cancer persist, and the incidence of some is even increasing. Nor can anyone claim the immediate prospect of a vaccine for Alzheimer's or diabetes. The death rate from heart disease may continue to decline, but we are still a long way from any dramatic decrease in its prevalence, its morbidity, or its costs. Both cancer and heart disease will long be with us because there are many, and different, kinds of both; there will never be a simple magic bullet for both, or at least that is highly unlikely.

There is also a logical problem with the chronic diseases of aging societies; some Europeans have come to call it the substitution problem, meaning the inevitable substitution of one potentially fatal disease in a person by another fatal disease. We will all die of something or other; if we don't die of cancer, our chances of dying from heart disease or Alzheimer's or kidney failure must correspondingly increase.[39]

Even if at the moment death rates in the United States for all age groups are declining, moreover, there is no reason to think that this can go on indefinitely. We have been glad, in the past, to be saved from death by one disease early in life in order to have the advantage of dying of another later in life. But the older we get, the shorter is the time between being saved from one disease and being killed by another. As two distinguished demographers have noted, "From the biological perspective . . . senescence is inevitable and progressive. This means that as progress is made against earlier-occurring disorders, those that emerge at later ages should be increasingly difficult to conquer."[40] We can shuffle the causes of death, and we can live longer in the process. But death is still waiting in hiding for all of us, eventually to make its appearance.

So far, I have put entirely to one side some very real possibilities for progress with chronic disease and disability: rehabilitation, prosthetics, palliation, and other means to help people better deal with their chronic disease. Progress here has been striking, as evidenced by elderly people whose mobility is preserved by hip replacements and whose ability to communicate is saved by hearing aids; by the extended survival time of cancer patients; by ingenious means of relieving chronic pain; and on and on. There is still considerable room for advancement here, and it will surely be pursued, though not inexpensively.

Yet from the evidence at hand, I conclude that there will mainly be palliative and rehabilitative victories over the leading chronic diseases for even the long foreseeable future. None of these diseases will be eradicated, and all will continue to take thousands of lives. In the diseases of aging, we seem to be up against some formidable biological barriers.

4. *Aging and the Compression of Morbidity.* Save for the cure of lethal disease, few dreams have captured the medical imagination so much as the compression of morbidity. Wouldn't it be wonderful, as Condorcet speculated over two centuries ago, if the sickness and decline that precede death in old age could be eliminated or radically reduced?[41] The compression of morbidity—the shortening of the period of illness prior to death—seems as intuitively plausible as it is attractive. Is this not the way nature seems to work with other animals, whose death is rarely preceded by a long period of decline? Is this not

a sensible goal for medicine, one that does not require us to invent a way to conquer death but only to overcome the sickness that precedes it?

But what is the evidence concerning the hoped-for compression of morbidity? It is at best mixed, tantalizing in some respects but far from sufficient to conclude that such compression is a certain future possibility. As developed by Dr. James Fries, its most serious proponent, the theory is that there will be a gradual compression of mortality around an average life expectancy of eighty-five, accompanied by a corresponding compression of morbidity.[42] The trouble here is that nature has been reluctant to play its assigned role. The evidence generally has shown that the longer people live, the more likely they are to experience illness and disability in their old age. Great effort has been expended to see if this trend, dominant for the past half century, shows any sign of a change. So far, the evidence to support such a change is weak.[43]

One reason, however, to hope that such a change might eventually appear is the possibility that the generally healthier lives that have been lived by the present generation of the elderly will begin to show themselves in the hoped-for compression. Some studies have shown not only a slight decline in disability in the elderly in recent years but also evidence that at least some elderly people, particularly those who have lived a healthy lifestyle in their earlier years, are less burdened by illness before their death than prior generations have been.[44]

There is no doubt that a significant compression of morbidity would make a great and beneficial difference in the lives of the elderly, and of course would equally promise a significant decline in the costs of their health and social care. But it is premature to conclude that such an era is near at hand. Some signs are promising, but they are hints only; and to make a decisive difference, the compression of morbidity must happen among many people, not only a fortunate few. If that is to come about, it will depend heavily upon a pattern of healthy behavior throughout a lifetime. In that respect, then, there is every reason to lead the kind of life that could make such hopes turn out to be true.

An obvious proviso needs at once to be added: compression of morbidity will only be possible if there is, at the end of life, no great rush to provide the kind of high-technology acute-care medicine—and even some forms of low-technology, ordinary medicine, such as antibiotics—that will extend the lives of sick people. A person could live a wholly healthy life until the optimally average eighty-five—the dream of compressed mortality—and then see enormous resources expended to keep him or her alive to eighty-six. In other words, the achievement of a compressed morbidity requires a medicine that has given up a goal now often pursued: that of artificially extending—even for the sake of some clear benefits—the period of decline and dying for the elderly. A sustainable medicine built around a compression of morbidity would aim to keep people healthy for as long as possible, then let them die with minimum technological intervention, even if it were potentially beneficial. Hence, the question to be considered is twofold: Could medicine find a way to achieve the compression of morbidity? And, if it could, would the culture be ready to accept the change in attitudes toward the extension of life necessary to make it work? We are still a long way from the first possibility, and probably no less distant from the second.

5. *Disease and the Genetic Revolution.* While medical researchers and the for-profit research industry are forever optimistic about the prospect of decisively curing disease, no excitement has quite matched that which genetic research has engendered. The claim in its behalf is sweeping and radical: genetic research and its clinical application promise to finally bring medicine to the root causes of disease. Once these causal, molecular mechanisms are understood, clinical medicine and medical technology will be in a superb position to eliminate many, if not most, of the deadliest diseases. "The premise of illness as an unpredictable casualty or Act of God,"

one enthusiast has written, "will be invalidated by genetic screening."[45] Of such enthusiasm, the biologist Robert Pollack has commented that "The fundamental premise of molecular biology—that any question about any living thing can be answered, and any disease understood and eradicated, by learning the detailed interactions of appropriate DNAs, RNAs, and proteins—has grown from an optimistic research strategy to the dominant agenda of a multibillion-dollar research juggernaut."[46] This juggernaut has been fueled by the belief that "the cure for all diseases would flow from an understanding of their molecular mechanisms."[47] Here, then, is the last biological obstacle: our genetic makeup at the molecular level.

How is the likely success of molecular medicine to be evaluated? The grandiose claims of some of its most ardent proponents must be approached warily: the raising of venture capital requires unrelenting optimism. The advance most hoped for is an understanding of the genetic foundations of disease, which may thus be combated at its core. The forerunner of this development, and the gateway to it, is the further improvement of what has come to be called predictive medicine—the ability to identify the likelihood of late-onset genetic, or genetically influenced, disease. "The 21st century [diagnostic] workup," one commentator has written, "may likely include a panel of DNA probes in place of a chemistry profile or complete cell count."[48]

There is still no way to evaluate properly these claims or hopes. They presume the possibility of an unprecedented domination of nature, and for just that reason it is hard to know how much credence to give them. Yet already there is no doubt that, through genetic counseling, screening, and prenatal diagnosis, a great deal of negative eugenics is already under way, involving the elimination—either through the avoidance of procreation or through abortion—of genetically defective babies. On the basis of progress so far, it is expected that these capabilities will increase. So also will the possibility of genetic therapy in utero as an alternative to abortion.[49]

Genetics and molecular medicine have made remarkable progress to date, but they have a long way to go before they come anywhere near the claims made in their behalf. Nor can it be known whether the genetic possibilities will be afford-able, genuine contributors to a sustainable medicine, rather than simply expensive add-ons. At the least, they remain only possibilities. The genetic revolution is still an idea—an inter-esting and important idea, but not yet far enough along for us to declare that it has found even in theory the answer to death, sickness, and aging. Genetically based diseases usually express themselves through environmental interactions, save for the less common single-gene anomalies. As P. A. Baird has re-minded us in a careful and balanced discussion of the genetic possibilities, "the simplistic model of disease causation that is currently present in our culture puts us at risk of foolish and precipitate action."[50] It is surely simplistic to expect that most diseases have simple genetic causes. While some direct ge-netic interventions will surely be possible, environmental in-terventions will probably be more important; and their development will be a complex and long-term task.

A New Era of Human Health?

I have called the five issues just discussed biological "ob-stacles" to progress. In each case, I am not saying there won't be gains in the future. Of course there will, and many of them. My contention is more moderate, but still stark: that there is no reasonable likelihood either that medical progress will usher in a dramatic new era of human health, or that there will be gains in the twenty-first century comparable to those made in the twentieth. The gains that medicine will achieve will be incre-mental, expensive, and erratically distributed among individu-als and groups rather than general in their impact. For some people, the benefits may be great; for most, less so. The reasons are that much of the easy progress has been accomplished and that the obstacles to further progress are exceedingly formidable. Death will not be conquered; average life expectancies will not gain an additional thirty or forty years. Infectious disease will not finally be eliminated, but will continue to plague human life. The chronic diseases of aging societies will not be conquered either, even if great progress is made in one or two—progress that will be offset by continued resistance among those that remain. There may well be some compression of morbidity among the elderly, but only if the next few decades see some dramatic improvement in living and health habits, changes that cannot be brought about by medical progress alone. For all the touting of a final genetic knockout of disease, there is no reason to expect such an event.

Naturally, I could be proved wrong in one or more of these predictions. But for there to be striking medical progress in the future—progress of a kind to radically improve population health—almost all the biological obstacles *together* would have to be overcome. The odds of such a massive development, on all major fronts, are relatively slight. Recall that the standard of assessment I have used to make this judgment, both in general and within each of the five categories, is whether the theoretical basis exists now for progress; whether the required research is already going on to make the progress feasible in the near term; and, finally, whether any of the research promises not only the hoped-for progress but also progress that would be consistent with a more sustainable medicine. None of those conditions are being met in general, even if one can find signs of such a possibility for a few diseases here and there.

The Costs of Pursuing the Dream

The argument of this book is that the costs—economic, social, and psychological—of relentlessly pursuing the hopeful dream of modern medicine *in an unaltered form* are no longer supportable. I stress "in an unaltered form" for two reasons. First, I wish to make clear that the original dream, played out—and still being played out—in what I earlier called the second historical era of medicine, was and is a noble and understandable dream, to which comparatively rapid and dramatic advances over the past century gave considerable credence. Second, I want to underscore the idea that it is not the fact that medicine has a dream that is the fatal flaw. Medicine ought to have a dream. It is the *form* that dream has taken that creates the problems.

Yet since most important human enterprises carry a price tag—nothing of value comes problem-free in this world—we might well ask, "So what?" So what if the modern quest for unending, open-ended medical progress carries with it high financial and human consequences? Isn't the real question whether those consequences are worth it, a decent trade-off given the gains and benefits achieved? Indeed, that is the right question, and the answer, I want to argue, is no. The consequences we now incur from contemporary progress as presently understood are not worth the gain we get. We can get a greater gain at a more affordable cost in other ways (a point I will develop later in the book). But what are those consequences? Let me discuss five—consequences that, if not taken seriously, will subvert the possibility of a sustainable medicine.

1. *An Escalating Economic Crisis in the Provision of Health Care.* One of the most remarkable developments of the past decade is the fact of economic stress in the provision of health care in almost every developed country. While he may have slightly overstated the matter, the observation in 1991 of Dr. Hiroshi Nakajima, director general of the World Health Organization, perfectly caught a general and worldwide trend: "The health system is deteriorating worldwide, in particular because of the continual rise in its prices, both in the rich countries and in the developing nations."[51] While the United

States has had the most publicized, notorious system—a nox-
ious combination of the most expensive and the least equitable—even countries with universal health care and lower
per capita costs began to run into problems by the end of the
1980s. On the surface, all looked well: countries with universal care managed to hold steady, for a number of years, the
percentage of their GNP devoted to health care—seemingly
in defiance of inflationary increases in other sectors. In great
part this was the result of government decisions not to allow
health care's share of the budget to increase, a policy that
helped wring out inefficiencies in many systems and controlled salaries and wages.

But not all was well below the surface, where the combination of aging societies, technological developments, and
public demand created shortages and widespread stress. By the
1990s, the early stability of costs had given way in many countries to relatively rapid annual percentage increases. Canada,
France, Germany, Japan, the United Kingdom, and the
United States all saw large increases in 1991–1992 after relative stability between 1980 and 1991.[52] Managed-care initiatives brought a quick drop in the rate of cost increase in the
United States by the end of the mid-1990s, but the persistence
of that drop is now in serious doubt. In response to these economic pressures in Europe, as well as to a weakening of the
welfare state, a variety of means to overtly or covertly ration
health care were introduced, together with a widespread privatizing of parts of many systems. Almost everywhere, there was
talk of a "crisis" in health care systems.

The universality of the economic pressures on health
care systems—regardless of the way they are organized and financed—points to a single, underlying cause beyond general
inflation: intensified use of expensive technological medicine,
coupled with increased demand, whether for individual or demographic reasons or both. While there are temporary lulls in
the upward pressure on medical costs, there is no good reason
to believe those costs can easily be controlled for long under

present health care systems.[53] We are, in short, seeing the economic consequences of the modern medical dream of constant progress—particularly the effort to overcome the biological obstacles I earlier described—and they are fearful. The dream can be pursued only by more rationing of health care, by forcing individuals to pay for more of their own care (often at the cost of other needs), or by nations spending an unwarranted and unwise portion of their resources on health care (as does the United States) and neglecting other goods critical to prosperous and humane societies.

2. *The Tyranny of Health, Risk, and Perfectionism.* The dream of modern medicine has had at least three profound effects on human consciousness. The first has been the instilling of a widespread belief that nothing more stands in the way of good health than an improved medicine and a decent, efficient health care system. The second effect has been increasingly to make all illness and disease seem to be a biological accident, one that can be avoided by better health care, better preventive screening, and better scientific knowledge. The third effect might be termed the encouragement of medical perfectionism, through crusades to eliminate all known sources of risk—fighting against what one writer has called a supposed risk epidemic—and all known causes of death and illness, reducing to zero the chance of death and injury, whether from accident or disease.[54] This risk-averse, perfectionist drive helps account for the growing gap between the actual state of people's health, actually improving for most, and their perceived situation, thought to be worsening. Despite the fact that people live, on the whole, healthier and longer lives than at any time in human history, and face fewer risks to health, they are more worried than ever about the dangers and less willing than ever to settle for something less than perfection.[55] The persistent difficulty of devising appropriate policies and practices for the end of life and the termination of treatment stands as an apt token of the problem of risk and perfectionism. More can always be

done, and there is often every incentive to do it. The old medical joke that a healthy person is someone who has not been adequately diagnosed is uncomfortably close to the truth.[56]

3. *Confusion Over the Proper Scope of Medicine.* There was a time when medicine was thought of use primarily to struggle against the natural ills that befall the body. That is no longer true. Not only is medicine increasingly drawn into the quest to serve individual desires and preferences having little if anything to do with health, it is now looked upon as a primary instrument to cope with social problems as well — most notably, of late, violence and substance abuse. Just as individual problems are increasingly medicalized — understood, that is, as problems that medicine can successfully treat — so also are many social problems. Medicine is looked to for help in getting at the "real" causes (e.g., genetic predispositions to violence) of those problems, or for help in cleaning up the results even if the causes lie in the social, not medical, realm (the relief of workplace stress, for instance).

The dream of modern medicine directly encourages this kind of thinking, in part by pointing to medicine's success in dealing with other human problems, and in part because it is so often imperialistically thought that a combination of better biological information and the power of clinical intervention can take on just about any human problem. The impulse that led the great eighteenth-century American physician Benjamin Rush to say that it would eventually "be as much the business of the physician as it is now of a divine to reclaim mankind from vice" is still alive and well.[57] An early sign of this syndrome (the only appropriate term for it) was in the history of the World Health Organization, founded just after the Second World War and motivated by a strong belief that better human health was the best way to avoid future wars — as if World War II stemmed from some kind of health problem![58] The fact that a social problem labeled as a "health" problem can usually command more public money is a significant contributing force as well. "Health" as a value sells better politically than "welfare."

4. *The Skewing of Medical Priorities.* The drive of modern medicine to save and extend life—at the core of ambitious progress—has been one of its great glories. At the same time, the pursuit of cure and the saving of life—the overwhelming priority given to the reduction of mortality—has meant a terrible neglect of the chronically ill, those who cannot be cured and who, over a long period of time, will die from their disease, or who will spend a life disabled as a result of it. Perhaps we have found the burden of personal care, the demands on patience and compassion, too high. The caring function of medicine, once its center, has been displaced to the sidelines. It is not a major source of money, prestige, or research awards. In the face of budgetary pressures, the care of the chronically ill of all ages—those who are proof against the miracles of medicine—has trouble gaining adequate support under managed care in the private sector, with long-term care for the elderly facing a particularly difficult future in the public sector, no longer even a subject for serious discussion in the fitful American debates on health care reform.

The priorities of research are equally skewed by placing the struggle against death first on the list (as has been the case for years at the National Institutes of Health); those of medical education are no less distorted when emphasis falls so heavily on the science of medicine and the use of technological interventions to cure illness. The net result is a medicine that, in the face of a rising burden of chronic disease and disability, still acts as if medicine is really nothing more than the pursuit of that form of progress satisfied only with making sick people well, not concerned with providing decent care to those beyond the reach of progress.

5. *The Health Care Gap Between Rich and Poor Nations.* The gap in health care expenditures, and in the quality of medi-

cine, between rich and poor nations is enormous. While that gap cannot be blamed on rich countries, the Western model of scientific medicine *has* widely captured the attention and the money of those in power in poor countries. Their physicians are often technologically trained, either in developed countries or in emulation of them.

The result is health systems that are often badly skewed in the direction of the same acute-care, technological model dominant in the developed countries. That is what medical progress is thought to be. Where the great need is for public health and primary care services, particularly in rural areas, there are instead advanced tertiary-care hospitals in the major cities. It is the dream of modern medicine that is responsible for this distortion, a dream that has been as contagious in poor as in rich countries. And if the modern medical dream has hardly created the gap between rich and poor nations by itself, it has surely exacerbated that gap and made it all the harder to introduce forms and models of medicine that would more directly meet the needs of the great majority of people.

At the same time as the gap between rich and poor nations persists, the steady introduction of expensive medical technologies is helping to open a gap between rich and poor in developed nations as well. The often rapid movement toward privatization in many developing countries (particularly in Latin America and Asia) is making its appearance in health care systems that were at one time comprehensive and equitable. A two-tier health care system is, in and of itself, not necessarily inequitable. If the basic health care guaranteed to all is relatively generous and decent, the fact that the wealthy can get something even better is not unjust. Only when a form of medicine emerges that makes it more and more difficult to incorporate the products of progress into the basic guaranteed health care system, and that forces more people to look to their strained private resources to pay for needed care, does progress itself become a problem. That is just the situation most countries are now moving toward, because of the rising cost of medical progress and the usually expensive remedies it offers.

Redefining "Progress"

The problematic character of the notion of progress, the real biological obstacles to its further playing out in the future, and the economic and human consequences of failing to acknowledge those obstacles, show that the long-standing faith in the idea of exuberant medical progress is severely flawed. The unlimited, expansionary progress sought by modern medicine—progress with no articulated or envisioned end and no well-reasoned priorities—is not a viable route to continued beneficial progress, nor does it supply an adequate basis for a future sustainable medicine. The idea of progress itself must now be redefined. In part this is because the present form of progress generates enormous, growing costs, over time returning comparatively less on investment in it. Furthermore, it as often as not fails to satisfy the expansive desire for improved health, which always outruns whatever level of health becomes available. A redefinition of progress is also needed because there has been considerable progress already. The baseline of knowledge and practice is now much higher than it was one hundred, fifty, even ten years ago. Where should we go from *here*, when we have already come so far?

Is there a better way of thinking about progress than medicine now entertains? The remainder of this book is devoted to sketching the outline of such an alternative, which requires rethinking our ideas of technological innovation, of nature, of the self and society. But it will be useful here to set the stage for that effort by briefly laying out a different way of thinking about progress.

In his provocative book *Frontiers of Illusion: Science, Technology, and the Politics of Progress*, Daniel Sarewitz has astutely shown the considerable gap between the quest for progress and the social benefits it actually delivers. Too often it is the quantity of progress that is celebrated, not its human impact. We should now set different standards of measurement for what we want to count as progress. The direction and distribution of progress should count, Sarewitz contends; not just its distance, and not just the accumulation of new knowledge and technological possibilities, but also their critical assessment and actual consequences.[59] That seems to me just right, and my own proposals are meant to embody the same spirit.

Four features of a possible alternative way of thinking about medical progress are worth identifying.

The first feature is that progress should be measured, on the whole, by changes in population health outcomes—that is, population death and illness rates. While the lives of individuals are clearly important—*my* life, and not just all of our lives together—measuring progress too heavily in individual, incrementalist terms will encourage indifference to the economic costs of that progress, to its overall benefit to society, and to the actual degree of advance being made. Our bias, that is, should be shifted in a population direction; though welcoming individual benefits, we must give them a secondary priority, if only because they rarely admit of limits or achieve full satisfaction. The main question should be: how is our collective, common health doing? The second feature of an alternative view of progress is stress on the need to reduce the perfectionism and risk aversion that mark the present expression of progress. The obsession with perfection and risk reduction encourages the development of expensive technologies benefiting comparatively few, or marginally helping many, just as it exacerbates the tension between what people want from medicine and what they are likely to get.

The third feature of an alternative notion of progress is that it will shift the focus from medical and technological improvements to amelioration of the social, economic, and cultural conditions that contribute so decisively to population and individual health. If the real goal of medicine is to improve health, then it will be crucial to take seriously all those circumstances that improve health, rather than to privilege the contributions medicine can make in achieving that goal. We need, that is, to take seriously a far broader view of the determinants of good health, finding ways to shift attention away from the supposed glamour of medical tactics and cures to and toward other, nonmedical strategies that might more directly and less expensively achieve the same ends.

The fourth feature of an alternative idea of progress is the most far-reaching: the alternative idea will not include the present intensive efforts to improve the health of those who have the greatest life expectancy in human history. This is to posit, in effect, at least one finite, final goal for medical progress to supplant its present goal-less, open-ended state. The average person in good health in the developed countries of the world (and living in a reasonably safe environment), *already* lives long enough to accomplish most reasonable human ends. A medicine that could assure those now being born that they could live as long—and only as long—and healthy lives as their parents should be perfectly acceptable. Neither the human species as a whole, nor most individuals, need more than the present average life expectancy in the developed countries (the mid-seventies to low eighties) for a perfectly satisfactory life. This ideal of a steady-state life expectancy at its present level would establish, happily, a finite and attainable goal: "Enough, already."

If "Enough, already" sufficed in the struggle with death, there would still be considerable room for beneficial progress. Advances in rehabilitation, health promotion and disease prevention, the compression of morbidity, and palliative care—all of which bear more on the quality than the quantity of life—would be valuable and welcome. To give them the highest priority would give due respect to the powerful biological obstacles to unlimited progress, would take better account of economic constraints, and would help deflate pressures for the marginal progress at the fringes of life that is now the most obvious consequence of medical efforts to combat mortality.

There will always be, at the frontiers of advancing progress, a ragged edge. By that image I mean to acknowledge the necessary and permanent gap between what medicine has already accomplished and what it might accomplish in the future.[60] No matter how far medicine goes, there will always be sick and suffering people on the ragged edge of progress. That edge will be different from era to era—the patients will have different problems—but it will always exist. If medicine believes that it must always advance to relieve illness and suffering, envisioning no criteria by which to decide that enough is enough, then the ragged edge of progress will always seem like a defeat of medicine and a goad to further progress. That is a mistaken way of thinking. The ragged edge can never be overcome, just moved.

A sustainable medicine requires, in sum, the acceptance of an idea of progress that sets finite goals, that is willing to accept adequacy rather than perfection, that tolerates a ragged edge, that has a sober respect for biological obstacles, and that understands the high human costs of an unwillingness to heed the limits to progress. Daniel Sarewitz is not far off the mark when he writes: "Political and cultural institutions might find their goals better served by responding to [their] problems as if scientific and technological progress had come to an end and the only recourse left to humanity was to depend upon itself."[61]

CHAPTER THREE

Sustainable Technology:
A Medical Oxymoron?

For all its maturity, the institution of medicine is not unlike a vulnerable child—new to the world, subject to the infections that beset the culture of which it is a part. Medicine has taken upon itself the struggle to overcome and dominate nature, a legacy of Baconian science. It has lent itself, sometimes willingly, sometimes not, to the market enterprise, seeking to find a way to turn human need into economic profit. It has often adapted to the protean self favored by contemporary life, resisting the notion of some overarching good and settling instead for those discrete biological goods that satisfy shifting individual needs and desires.

Practically none of that adaptation would be possible, however, if medicine did not have at its disposal the possibility of constant technological innovation and an abiding faith in the idea of progress. Technological innovation is the most practical expression of the idea of progress. Medical innovation is the application of scientific knowledge to obtain usable techniques, methodologies, and tools to improve the practice of medicine, and thereby to improve health. Of course, it is obvious that medical innovation can aim not simply at health but also at achieving personal goals that may have little directly to do with health.

Technological Innovation: A Second Chance Against Nature?

Easy though it is to find countless utopians who envision the conquest of biology by medicine, the greater challenge to a sustainable medicine may lie with those who hold out more modest, but still potent, expectations. Consider some of the claims made in behalf of medical innovation. "Medical Community Must Get the Message That It Is a Key Player in US Economic Growth," read a headline in the newsletter of Research America, described as an "Alliance for Discoveries in Health."[1] "Only innovation can enable the dramatic and sustained cost reductions required for successful health care reform," wrote three experts in the journal *Science*.[2] The Health Care Technology Institute, supported by the medical technology industries, prophesies that innovation will bring a great reduction of disease through preventive medicine at one extreme and home-based personal medicine at the other.[3] Dr. Harold Varmus, director of the National Institutes of Health, foresees the day when a "brilliant young neuroscientist" will see a route to the cure of Alzheimer's disease through an anti-Alzheimer's drug to be developed by a biotechnology company.[4] A *Wall Street Journal* headline in 1994, expressing concern that health care rationing could hurt pharmaceutical research, proclaimed that "Killing Drug Research Kills People."[5]

Innovation, in short, is profitable, cost-reducing, the best opponent of disease, and a moral requirement.[6] There is truth in these claims, but how much truth? No doubt the potential for innovation is great, particularly if the standard of success is incremental gain. Dr. William Schwartz, a physician and shrewd policy analyst, has listed a number of the likely possibilities—ranging from better-targeted drugs with fewer side effects, to better ways to fight autoimmune diseases such as arthritis, to assorted genetic therapies, to means of screening for cancer—and it is possible, almost every week, to find some innovation being celebrated.[7] In 1994, the Health Care Technology Institute provided a list of emerging technologies for some chronic diseases: transmyocardial laser revascularization for ischemic heart disease; noninvasive blood glucose monitoring for diabetes; tissue engineering for bone and cartilage disorders; ultrasonic ablation for prostate cancer; and fluorescent endoscopy for lung cancer.[8]

Such advances surely help explain, if explanation is even needed, the powerful attraction of developing new technologies. Yet the attraction of technology does not lie simply in its actual or potential effectiveness. Technology has other uses as well—economic, social, and psychological—uses that overshadow or obscure its actual effectiveness and make the latter of less consequence than strict medical logic would seem to require. There are at least three domains in which technological innovation is powerfully alluring; they are mutually reinforcing but individually identifiable.

1. *Clinical Attractions.* If medicine cannot beat biology all the way down, the next best strategy is to nibble away at it; this, medical technology does exceedingly well. Physicians are trained to use technology, to depend upon it, and to want ever-improved technology. The astute physician Eric Cassell has nicely described the attraction of technology for practicing clinicians. It plays to their sense of *wonder*—the possibility of knowing so much about, and doing so much to, the human body. It offers the lure of the *immediate*—"the numbers of the readout, images on film, dexterity required for its deployment,

technical complexities, tubes, wires, plugs . . . and on and on exist in the here and now—the immediate moment."[9] The pull of the immediate is nicely complemented by the lure of the *unambiguous*: "More sophisticated means less ambiguous; the better the piece of equipment, the clearer the values."[10] Unambiguousness leads to its sibling, *certainty*: "Whatever technique promises greatest certainty, even if inappropriate, will diminish the use of techniques associated with greater uncertainty."[11] The chase after certainty plays easily into the hands of another great attraction of technology, that of the (self-perpetuating) *power* it puts in the hands of physicians.

To Cassell's list of clinical attractions, I would add two more, the pursuit of *perfection* and *risk reduction*, which I touched upon in the previous chapter. Technology offers a seemingly effective way to deal with risk, of central importance in a medicine that has a potent streak of perfectionism running through it. Risk is reduced by good diagnosis and screening, and is no less effectively identified by those means. Prenatal screening, initially introduced in the 1960s to help women most at risk of fetal abnormalities, is now a standard part of pregnancy care for all women. Ultrasound, for instance, was once rarely used; it is now routine. The pursuit of risk reduction through screening for cancer and other conditions is already a major medical effort. Medical perfectionism is an offshoot of the general drive for progress: every beneficial medical outcome now possible can be further improved, and every lingering problem reduced or overcome—rehabilitation to jog again, not just to walk. The idea of partial success as a long-term goal is anathema: the tacit point is, inch by innovative inch, to rid ourselves of *all* sickness and disease. The field of pediatrics is a perfect example: the fact that children are remarkably healthier than in earlier times, and far more likely to survive their childhood, has not led to the withering of pediatrics as a medical field. Pediatrics has simply raised its standards, pursued all known risks, rejected all fatalism: it will not in its ideals accept even slightly unhealthy children. In a world where the pressures are all toward the one- or two-child family, moreover, economic and social forces exacerbate those tendencies. Much more is invested in fewer children; illness, much less death, with those children is simply not tolerable.

2. *Public Demand.* It would be a mistake to believe that technological innovation attracts only physicians. The public wants the goods of technology just as much. People want their doctors to have the power to cure illness, to be confident in their treatments, to have good machines and gauges and tubes to rely upon for precise results. They also believe that technological innovation is precisely what promises those goods. Clinical perfectionism on the part of physicians finds its ideal partner in the perfectionism of the public.

People who are sick go to doctors for help. They want something to be done to them that will make them better, and they look as much to the doctor's tests and devices as to the doctor's knowledge. Medical technology is scientific knowledge incarnate and a visible sign that efforts are being made to respond to patient needs. Words and touch can often have the same effect, but modern medicine has managed to convey the message that the way to move beyond nice words to efficacious deeds is technology. That is something patients can see for themselves: the pill relieves their pain; the operation allows them to walk again; the screening test picks up the condition of which they were unaware; sophisticated information systems move their medical records about at a rapid speed. People who live in a world dominated by technology, at home and at work, expect the same in their medical care, and the technology of medicine is among the most touted of all. Indeed, medical technology is primary, for it keeps us alive and well so we can use the other technologies.

3. *The Market.* Medical technology is the result, in part, of government-supported research. But most technological innovation comes about as a commercial venture, the effort of

some company to create a product that will be purchased and used by doctors, hospitals, and clinics and duly appreciated by patients.

Medicine has been an enormously profitable industry. There is, however, no growth of profits in a steady-state medical technology. Patents eventually run out, some drugs cease to be effective, and generic drugs no longer covered by patent protection bring poor profit. Technologies must change, improve, do something a little different and a little better to be a source of assured increased profits. Innovation is not just clinically exciting, then; it is the key and necessary ingredient in generating ongoing profit. Pharmaceutical companies and the manufacturers of medical equipment must constantly innovate. Their competitors force them to do so, the doctors always want something better, the public is ready to pay for improvement, and technological innovation in and of itself is a source of pride and satisfaction for the innovators. The results have been impressive: a steady flow of new and improved technologies, pleasing to doctors, researchers, and patients alike.

The market also works most effectively with that view of the self and society which eschews overarching moral and philosophical meaning and value. This view places the emphasis instead on the satisfying of individual wants and preferences, including but also going beyond people's very real need to avoid death and to stay well and functioning. The market as an economic ideology and set of techniques encourages us to move beyond a medicine that is rooted in its own history and traditions and oriented to some objective standard of health, to a medicine that is simply a collection of knowledge and techniques, to be used and exploited as anyone sees fit. The market exploits that proclivity most effectively.

As John Powles noted over twenty-five years ago, "To an increasing extent medical technology is serving as a mask for non-technical functions. . . . The more attention within medicine is focused on the technical mastery of disease, the larger become the symbolic and non-technical functions of that

89

technology."[12] Technological innovation is full of hope, money, and enough medical successes to sustain confidence that we are on the right track. All of those features move it into the symbolic realm, serving functions of which health is only one.

Can Technological Innovation Be Made Affordable?

None of this might matter in the least if the technologies developed can be made affordable. Then we would have a sustainable medicine, one that simultaneously gratified all desires and met all needs: the best of all possible worlds. But can medical technology be affordable? Some say yes, others say no. Or is that even the right question? To phrase the question usefully is difficult. Do we want to know if technology is, in principle, in theory, affordable? Or do we want to know if it is likely in practice to be affordable? There is another reason as well for the difficulty of the question: almost anything will be thought affordable if we consider it important enough for our life or welfare. Nations threatened with invasion always find self-defense affordable, however poor they might be.

I will not try here to parse the many different ways the question of affordability might be posed and approached. My own view is that medical technology will be affordable if it satisfies two conditions. First, within medicine, no one technology or set of technologies for one group of patients should threaten the medical needs of other patients. This means that we must carefully consider any technological innovation, asking what the opportunity costs of the technology are (that is, comparing alternative ways the same money might be spent to improve health and considering to what extent the innovation might require the diversion of funds already helping other patients). Second, the pursuit of medical innovation should not seriously threaten other important social needs.

90

Another stipulation is necessary. The most plausible way of evaluating the economic implications of technological innovation is by examining the trends revealed in the historical record. That is the only available method for evaluating whether *claims* that more research and technological innovation will control or reduce health care costs are likely to prove true—for instance, will improved cancer therapies or hypertension drugs save money in the long run? Have similar innovations done so in the past? I want, moreover, to specify that it is the *aggregate affordability* of technological innovation that should concern us, not only the affordability of this or that particular technology. No *single* technological innovation, or widely distributed discrete technology, could possibly sink us financially. It is all of them *together* that pose the more complex problem. It is all too easy to make affordability seem feasible by focusing on the success stories, or by singling out individual technologies and touting the benefits they provide; this can seduce us into thinking that a particular benefit, even if expensive, is well worth it and in any case not by itself a great contributor to overall cost increases.

It is perfectly true that kidney dialysis taken by itself is a drop in the overall bucket of health care costs, as is the drug clozapine for schizophrenia, or AZT and protease inhibitors for HIV disease, or tPA for thromboembolytic clots. Put together, however, they tell a different story. Their combined costs are huge. That is the story that concerns me here, for my question is not whether some innovations can be affordable—to which the answer is certainly yes—but whether unlimited technological innovation in the aggregate at the present pace is affordable. To that, my answer is no. Since 1960, technology costs per capita have increased by 791 percent, compared with an increase of 269 percent for health care spending as a percent of gross national product. The costs of technology were, by far, the most significant source of increased health care costs during recent decades.[13]

Both historical evidence and recent trends suggest that

91

constant and unlimited innovation at the present level is not indefinitely affordable, and there is no evidence of any consequence to suggest a likely change in that pattern. What kind of evidence would that have to be? Very simply, it would have to show that technological innovation *in general* tends to lower or stabilize costs. Unfortunately, the evidence points in exactly the opposite direction. Innovative technologies in the aggregate raise costs. It is not difficult to understand why when the dynamic of innovation is examined.

Why Is Unlimited Technological Innovation Unaffordable?

Four general economic phenomena have dominated the process of recent technological innovation in societies that already have a well-advanced state of good health, many long-established technologies, aging populations, and a general control of infectious disease. These phenomena are (1) the relationship between cost and overall use of a technology; (2) the expansion of diagnostic and therapeutic possibilities; (3) the tendency toward a duplication of technologies; and (4) the increased costs of postponing death.

1. Unit Cost Down, Overall Use Up. It is often argued that, with improvement, the initial (often high) unit cost of new technologies will drop dramatically, thus putting them within wider reach. That is surely correct, as everything from television sets to computers to dialysis machines shows. But less noted (though surely known) is that the drop in individual unit cost is exactly what opens the door to exceedingly high aggregate costs: the cheaper a device or procedure, the more people can afford it. As a society, we spend far more total money on computers now, when a PC is inexpensive, than we did on earlier, expensive ones. The unit costs of bypass surgery, dialysis, and diagnostic scanning have dropped significantly over the years, but as a direct result the total number of such procedures and their overall costs have increased enormously.[14]

2. *More Diagnostic and Treatment Possibilities.* A great attraction of technological innovation is that it provides new and sometimes more effective means of diagnosis and treatment. Yet both tend to increase health care costs. Clearly, if no diagnosis at all was earlier available, a whole new cost is added by the innovation. Genetic screening for breast cancer is a recent example, stimulated by the increased possibility of detecting a genetic predisposition to the disease.[15] The same is true of new treatments: when nothing could be done, no costs were incurred. When we extend the range of diagnosis and treatment into new territory, costs must and will go up.

The new techniques of genetic screening for breast cancer come on top of the rapidly increasing use of expensive bone marrow transplantation for its treatment, by no means yet supported by good evidence of its efficacy. As the economist Joseph Weisbrod has noted, while some technologies reduce costs (a polio vaccine or drug treatments in place of expensive ulcer surgery), "most technological advances in recent years have not been cost reducing. . . . Rather than substituting for even more costly measures, they have provided additional ways to save life or to detect problems that then require costly treatment. These new technologies have much to commend them, but cost reduction is not one of them."[16]

3. *Technological Duplication and Add-ons.* The historical record of late indicates that new diagnostic procedures rarely displace the older ones—especially if the latter are still perceived to have some value, as is almost always the case. The quest for added clinical certainty, the obsession with risk reduction and medical perfectionism, means that new technologies are often used in addition to, not as substitutes for, the older technologies. The older devices may continue to provide information not available from the newer ones, even if the lat-

ter add something not supplied by the former. The history of diagnostic scanning devices, which has seen X rays supplemented by numerous other devices—CT scans, PET scans, and MRIs—is a good illustration of this phenomenon. Most hospitals will have more than one such device, and some will have all of them.[17]

4. *Saving Life and Increasing Costs.* When new diagnostic and therapeutic options emerge that save life, they necessarily create a new level of costs, however beneficial we may judge them. We will now have two costs on our hands: the cost of the treatment that saves a life now, and the cost of whatever subsequent condition will eventually kill the patient—the costs, that is, of what I have elsewhere called the "twice cured, once dead" phenomenon.[18] The cost of death is deferred to a later illness, while in the meantime we must pay for the successful treatment that makes the deferral possible. When, in addition, the explicit goal is to advance progress and thus to "improve the quality of care"—the great rallying cry for innovation—costs will and must go up.[19] As the Health Insurance Association of America showed almost a decade ago, in recent years most new technologies—some 80 percent—have increased, not decreased, costs.[20] Among the twenty-nine new technologies they listed as increasing costs were implantable defibrillators, advances in pacemakers, bone growth stimulators, penile prostheses, implantable infusion pumps, Doppler ultrasound, MRIs, PET scanners, liver transplants, and infection control for AIDS. Only six technologies, among them valvuloplasty, automated clinical chemical analyzers, endoscopic lasers, and peripheral vascular angioplasty, were listed as decreasing costs. Now it well might be objected that, even if correct, this list was generated ten years ago. Perhaps there has been a change in direction since then. I have, however, been unable to uncover any current information to indicate any significant shift toward cost-reducing technologies. Given what might be called its economic logic, medical innovation adds new possibilities of diag-

nosis and treatment, possibilities that did not previously exist. It is hardly any wonder they tend, on the whole, to increase rather than decrease costs in the aggregate.

We will have to choose between improving quality by constant innovation and controlling costs. We cannot have it both ways. Technological innovation remains an inherent source of increased costs, a factor as evident in the realm of medicine as it is in the cost of automobiles, airplanes, housing, or information technology.

Technology and Outcome Assessment

The obvious force of technological innovation in increasing costs has led to one important response. What has come to be called "evidence-based medicine" has the aim of carefully and scientifically assessing both old and new technologies for their clinical utility and cost-effectiveness, and sometimes for their cost-benefit ratio. With that information in hand, hospitals and clinics will, in theory, be able to better judge which technologies to procure, how best to use those they already have, and how to calculate the costs and benefits of innovation. Practice guidelines for physicians can also be developed that will foster a frugal and prudent use of technology. Evidence-based medicine is a splendid idea in its aspirations and hard to resist as a general strategy. In many cases, it has already succeeded in leading to a more defensible, economical use of technology, if only by focusing attention on the issue of efficacy. It has led to a reduction in the length of hospital stays, to the elimination of some useless procedures, and to a finer appreciation of the circumstances under which one procedure rather than another should be used (for example, angioplasty versus bypass surgery).[21]

Problems arise, however, when technology assessment is offered as a clean and simple panacea for the problem of the use of technology as well as for technological innovation. It can only be depended upon in a limited way to make a real difference—a difference well worth pursuing, but fatally flawed as a way to escape the problems of technology. For technology assessment has its own weaknesses.

Costs and Difficulties of Adequate Assessment. Good technology and outcome assessment is expensive and time-consuming. Only a small portion of existing technologies, not to mention the constant stream of new ones, can be assessed in a scientifically sound way.[22] The effort to compare two thromboembolytic—clot-dissolving—therapies, tPA and streptokinase, consumed many years, generated much controversy, and cost millions of dollars. It was financed by a company, Genentech, that had a financial stake in the outcome, creating some (mainly unfair) doubt about the results. Yet without the commercial support, the study might not have been carried out at all; and no equally extensive and expensive study is likely to be mounted to clarify the results. In some cases—to test, for example, the effectiveness of bone marrow transplantation for women with disseminated breast cancer—efforts have floundered because of the difficulty of recruiting subjects for a scientifically valid study; the search for cures and treatments for HIV disease has had the same kinds of problems. Given the expenses and difficulties of solid technology assessment, it has been necessary to set some priorities, and to settle for less than ideal scientific validity.[23]

Ambiguous Outcomes. From the first, the outcome assessment movement has been plagued by what might be called the yes or no dream: that it will be possible to come up with a definitive, scientifically based judgment on the effectiveness of a treatment or on the indications warranting the use of a diagnostic procedure. The reality has been otherwise. The results of many if not most studies are ambiguous and probabilistic. They are ambiguous, in the sense that they may not point to an obvious and definitive conclusion, but rather to an "it all depends" assessment: in some cases the procedure studied is a useful procedure, in other cases not, and in still others perhaps yes and perhaps no. (This was the result of the controversy over mammograms for women between forty and fifty.) The results are probabilistic in that they provide general odds on clinical effectiveness, but no way of telling what those odds mean for a particular patient.[24] This is the standard problem with all medical probabilities, and it is why medical decisions for individual patients necessarily remain full of uncertainty, even with good general data in hand. Cost-effectiveness is hardly less complicated, and raises many comparable questions concerning individual, as distinguished from general, benefits.[25]

However hard it has been to get good effectiveness studies, it is even more difficult to get good cost-benefit results.[26] The case of tPA versus streptokinase can be cited again. The Genentech study did find a slight (1 percent) reduction in death rates when tPA is used after a heart attack, but at some increased risk of a brain hemorrhage and at a considerably increased cost over streptokinase ($2,500 versus $600). It is good to have this information and this assessment, but it hardly tells us how physicians should act. Whether a 1 percent reduction in risk of death, but with increased side hazards and at a high cost, is "worth it" or not is a moral and economic question, not to be answered by the medical data alone or by better data. This is how it will be with most assessed technologies, save in those increasingly rare cases where some technology is hardly effective at all. When life is at stake, a statistically unlikely outcome can still look better than the alternative.

Onetime Savings. To the extent that ineffective or non-cost-beneficial technologies are a major part of our health care problems, outcome assessment seems necessary and valuable. But William Schwartz has effectively argued that to cut waste from the health care system will produce a onetime savings only, driving costs down for a time, but only for a time. That seems to be exactly what has happened with managed care.

97

New technologies yet to be assessed, as well as other factors, will just drive up costs once again, but the next time without the benefit of further fat to be eliminated.[27]

Moral and Legal Problems. It quickly became evident that physicians would resist outcome assessments and outcome guidelines, particularly if the latter are made mandatory. The physicians' worry (though only in the United States) is in part legal: they fear being sued for not conducting some additional tests or for not using treatments they found doubtful, whatever the available data might say. A more significant objection is that, because of the uncertainties in treating individual patients and the probabilistic nature of the data, physicians should never be bound by rigid treatment and technology-limitation rules—that is, forced to practice "cookbook medicine."[28] They should also not be forced to set aside their own clinical experience and the experience of those clinicians whom they admire.

Medicine remains as much an art as a science, and to ask physicians to conform rigidly to outcome assessments would be both morally offensive to their professional integrity and a hazard to patients. The fact that the courts have shown a steady and consistent readiness to set aside outcome studies and insurance reimbursement restrictions in favor of physician and patient choice has further undercut the force of outcome assessments.

Outcome Assessment and Economic Incentives. Nonetheless, despite physician resistance, the managed-care movement in the United States is demonstrating that doctors will change their diagnostic and treatment behavior if there are sufficient economic and other incentives to force them to do so.[29] The threat of losing patients for failure to follow practice guidelines or treat patients within a range of practices considered acceptable can be effective. It may well be that outcome assessment will not, in the end, work unless tied to economic rewards and punishments. Naturally, this is not a situation to warm the hearts of physicians *or* patients; it threatens many values long taken for granted in the way doctors treat patients and were trained (in another era) to treat them. At the same time, if guidelines are based on valid evidence, such incentives would seem appropriate enough, however distasteful.

Effectiveness and Affordability. Perhaps the most general error that has pervaded the outcome assessment movement is the assumption that if a treatment can be shown to be effective, it ought to be given to patients. But there is, unhappily, no necessary correlation at all between individually effective treatment and socially affordable treatment. It is an old story: what's good for you or me may not be good for the community as a whole. It is a mistake to assume that effectiveness is equivalent to affordability. These are totally separate issues. The most serious problems of medical technology and innovation come from effective but expensive treatments, especially those that are expensive in the aggregate. Insofar as medical research can develop more effective treatments, to that extent will our economic and moral problem become worse, not better. This is a classic, still-valid instance of the problems of success.

Now nothing I have said about outcome assessment should be taken as opposition to its use. On the contrary, it is exceedingly important and can use all the resources it can get; and it should get more. I only want to indicate that outcome assessment cannot, and will not, by itself, deal with the problems and costs of technology and technological innovation.

Pathologies of Hope

There are three likely responses to the mainly pessimistic line of argument about medical innovation that I have laid out here, all of them familiar to anyone who follows the literature of health policy, of biomedicine, or of medical progress. All offer a far more optimistic view of the future than I have, none propose a new, sustainable model for the technological medicine of the future, and all propose that with organizational reform, better outcome assessment, or the fruits of future research and innovation, can overcome the present range of problems. I call these responses "pathologies of hope" to indicate how they trade heavily on an indomitable hope that future solutions to current problems will in fact be found, and to suggest that the hope is pathological in that no present negative evidence is allowed to contradict it.

This pathological hope is the extreme form of a faith in progress that will not be dampened by contradictory evidence. The Enlightenment idea of progress and innovation in its late-twentieth-century manifestation is perfectly capable of digesting failure—and then calling for still more progress to correct it, progress that, it is doggedly believed, would inevitably come if given a chance. The pathologies of hope help to explain, in the biomedical context, what Christopher Lasch described as the puzzling "resilience of progressive ideology in the face of discouraging events that have shattered the illusion of utopia."[30] Medical pathologies of hope trade in assumptions about the efficacy of improved management, the benefits of new biological knowledge, and the power of technological innovation to overcome obstacles. Sometimes these assumptions are invoked alone and sometimes in combination.

1. *Managerial Miracles.* The first pathology insists that the root of the problem lies not in the expanding use or growing catalogue of medical technologies, but in poor management.

The abiding faith of an economic and managerial perspective is that, with clever organization and greater efficiency, a decent level of health care can be provided in all but the poorest societies. The liberal version of this perspective places its trust in good government planning and controls, whether centralized or decentralized, and it is geared to the available level of public economic support for health care. This version is by no means incompatible with both patient and physician discretion, but in the end it looks to government to establish the economic framework and to provide overall management and cost control. The conservative version of the managerial perspective places its faith in the power of the market, specifically in the ability of competition to enforce efficiency and hold down costs, and in economic incentives and disincentives to shape individual consumption and provider provision of health care resources. It rejects centralized government management.

Despite the fact of stress in every health care system, *however that system is organized* (and it is rare now to see a system that is either purely government-controlled or purely market-driven), health policy analysts and policymakers almost never question the goals of modern medicine or the sacred dogmas of progress and innovation. The resulting managerial and economic perspective on medicine and health care is, in the end, either indifferent to or agnostic about what medicine should try to do or what a health care system should try to bring to people. The abiding conviction is that, *whatever the goals of medicine may be* (a political or moral issue, not an organizational one), an organizational solution can be found to embody them. Yet the evidence of problems in every health care system these days casts a deep shadow on that faith. Few if any countries have developed a satisfying way to manage and finance contemporary health care systems. None have discovered how to well manage the costs of new, beneficial, and widely desired technologies.

2. *Salvation Through Research.* The second pathology of hope rests on the belief that the ultimate source of medical progress lies in deeper and better basic biological and biomedical knowledge. The stress on basic knowledge can be seen in a number of areas and in the soaring, unlimited hopes they spawn. For many these days, molecular biology holds the key

101

to genetic influences on disease and health, and thus provides the royal road to the complete eradication of disease. For some researchers, the key to the conquest of nature lies in a better understanding of the immune system. For psychiatric researchers of late, the way to the mastery of mental illness, to the solution of the ancient puzzle of the relationship between mind and body, lies in grasping the organic, neurological basis of mental disease.

Like faith in managerial efficacy, belief in research proceeds without much attention to the possibility that there may be basic biological impediments to an ultimate understanding and control of disease, or to the possibility that technological innovation growing out of fundamental research will rapidly add to the costs of care. What Renée C. Fox has referred to as the "ritualized optimism" of clinical research in the "therapeutic innovation cycle" is a direct outcome of the belief in progress—whatever the counterevidence. The war against cancer—with its incremental, costly, and often only marginally beneficial new treatments—is perhaps the most striking illustration of the persistence of this belief. "Periodically," Fox writes, "it is announced that an agent has been discovered that has the potential to eliminate primary tumors and to slow the growth and prevent the spread of metastatic tumors. . . . [There follow] more cautiously phrased and soberly toned publications . . . and this sets in motion once more, the same therapeutic innovation cycle."[31]

3. *The Promise of Technological Innovation.* Within modern medicine there has been a long-standing, if usually tacit, struggle between those who bet on basic biomedical knowledge as the certain way to the control or conquest of disease, and those who look to technological innovation—the third pathology of hope. The two bets are by no means incompatible. But they move in different directions and have behind them different driving forces. For those who believe in technological innovation, what counts is the success of a drug or machine or other

therapy in achieving a desired result, whether cure or amelioration. Technological innovation carries on the old tradition of looking for what works, with a relative indifference to the basic biology underlying its success.

The modern medical-industrial complex in particular, made up of the pharmaceutical and medical-devices industries most notably, looks to technological innovation to generate "fast, effective relief" of illness and at the same time provide high profits. The industry's contention is that innovation can provide medical relief even in the absence of full biological understanding, and that innovation is the most promising way to control health care costs: cheaper and more effective diagnostic and therapeutic modalities can, with a greater R & D investment, be found. But as I have tried to show in this chapter, the claim that treatments that are both generally cheaper *and* more effective are in the offing has no evidence to support it.

Does Medicine Do Any Good?

I have tried to show that there are both formidable difficulties in the way of affordable technological innovation and an unfortunately well-developed defense system against acknowledging those difficulties. A question must now be asked: does modern medicine do any good? Since a considerable, even overwhelming portion of the health benefits attributed to medicine stem from technological innovation, it is important to know whether there *has* been improved health traceable to medicine. Does medically based, ever-changing technological care make a difference? The unambiguous answer is, well, yes and no. Yes, technology obviously makes a difference at the margins of life: it increases life expectancies, reduces many forms of morbidity, helps in the palliative and rehabilitative care of large numbers of patients.

There is good evidence to show, for example, that medicine does contribute to a lowering of death rates, and in all age groups.[32] The decrease in cancer death rates in children, the increased survival time of all cancer victims, and the increase in life expectancy beyond the age of seventy-five show the impact of modern medicine and technological sophistication, to mention only three obvious examples. Organ transplantation, kidney dialysis, open-heart surgery, and a wide array of drugs save lives. Immunization programs, the fruit of biomedical research, are an obvious triumph of scientific medicine. Perhaps even more important, and usually overlooked by the sharpest critics of medicine, have been the improvements in caring for those with disease, when cure is not possible: the vast number of people whose pain can more effectively be relieved, or the handicapped who can now be helped with rehabilitation, or the mentally ill who can be better enabled by psychoactive drugs to cope with life. These are improvements in the quality of life, though not necessarily or usually its length.

Yet however important these contributions, they are not equivalent to a sustainable medicine, nor do they show that medicine's contribution to health is at all proportionate to its costs, or that the same gains might not have been achieved by nonmedical means, at least in part. The problem noted presciently by John Powles twenty-five years ago is, if anything, more pronounced now: "Medicine," Powles wrote, "contains its own particular expression of the wider crisis—diminishing returns and a self-defeating dependence on economic growth to solve the health problems associated with such growth."[33] And a decade ago Dr. William B. Schwartz came to an even starker judgment: "The long-term control of the rate of expenditures . . . requires that we curb the development of *clinically useful* technology."[34]

But the second half of the answer to the question whether medicine makes a difference is no, not all that much, if the health of the population as a whole is considered. As Theodore Marmor and his colleagues have noted,

"Some of the best kept secrets of longevity and good health are to be found in one's social, economic, and cultural circumstances."[35] While it is not quite accurate to call it a secret, this conclusion squarely fits the facts. Medical historians and epidemiologists are fond of noting that the great twentieth-century increase in life expectancy began to manifest itself in the last half of the nineteenth century, when death rates began to decline well before medicine could make any difference.[36] The reduction in infant mortality rates—which until very recently were the principal determinant of average life expectancy—came about mainly as the result of better nutrition and sanitation, not medical care.

To be sure, once technological medicine had taken hold—beginning with the advent of antibiotics in the 1930s and 1940s, together with many other advances—it did strengthen the trend toward increased life expectancy, particularly for the elderly, that was already under way. Still, not only has there been a relatively slight decline in death rates since 1950, estimated at 6 percent, it also seems true, as one important analysis has shown, that by the 1970s the "early and dramatic improvements in health status resulting from medical interventions were not repeated."[37]

As the distinguished Canadian health economists Robert G. Evans and G. L. Stoddard have noted, "It is not that no [health] needs remain, that the populations of modern societies have reached a state of optimum health. This is obviously not the case. Nor is it claimed that medicine has had no effect on health. This too is clearly false. The concern is rather that the remaining shortfalls, the continuing burden of illness, disability, distress, and premature death, are less and less sensitive to further extensions in health *care*. We are reaching the limits of medicine."[38] Moreover, Evans and Stoddard add, "overexpansion of the health care system can in principle have negative effects not only on the well-being of the population, but even on its *health*. . . . A society that spends so much on health care that it cannot or will not spend adequately on other health-*

enhancing activities may actually be reducing the health of its population [italics in original]."[39]

Medical technology does bring about comparatively small incremental gains for most people, and some dramatic gains for others (organ transplant recipients, for instance). But for everyone the gains are usually now achieved at a relatively high and increasing cost, with little effect on general population health, and they are usually not equally or even fairly distributed. This broad truth is easily obscured by the dazzle of technology. Physicians and patients want it to work, each for their own reasons. Those who invent and sell the medical technology want it to work as well. Medical innovation, in a dynamic that draws on the values of the culture, moves ahead and will likely continue to move ahead even in the face of open and full knowledge that social and public health forces are what make the greatest and final difference to population health.

Precisely because medical innovation is both exciting and possible, the source of economic as well as psychological profit, it is far easier to pursue culturally than social and public health innovation. A decisive cure for cancer, which is not likely to appear soon, is nonetheless far more likely than a decisive change in the effect of class and education on health status; to produce that is a real challenge.

Rethinking Progress and Innovation

So far, I have tried to show that the dominant view of progress and technological innovation—unlimited in its speculative possibilities—cannot realistically be sustained in the face of biological fact. If there are no inherent limits to the human capacity to overcome biology—and that would be impossible to demonstrate—there are clearly a number of emerging de facto limits and exceedingly high, perhaps economically impassable, mountains, not unlike the practical limits to exploring outer space. The conviction that technological innovation is the best way to pursue improved and cost-effective health does not offer a viable course for the future. It cannot produce a sustainable medicine. It can only guarantee an endless financial, social, and psychological struggle.

The trouble in trying to make that point persuasive, however, is that most people, both inside and outside the medical community, still believe in technological innovation and the gains it can bring. Even if they worry about the cost of it all, they have been reassured by an army of scientific optimists and efficiency experts that all will soon be well—if not tomorrow, then the next day. It is not sufficient to challenge such a belief system—expansive, inclusive, ever-hopeful, and ambitious—with evidence that it is not working now and will not, cannot, work in the future. Its proponents can always charge its critics with undue pessimism, inborn Ludditism, and—if all else fails—a willful turning of their backs on a sea of human suffering that only zeal, faith, research, and more progress can ultimately relieve.

The only good defense against these objections is to present an alternative vision of progress and medical innovation that can capture the imagination as effectively as the present no longer supportable but deeply ingrained one.

Sustainable Innovation

At the end of the last chapter I proposed four alternative ways of thinking about medical progress for the future: a focus on population, not individual, health improvement; a reduction of the drive toward total risk reduction and medical perfectionism; a focus on improving those background social, economic, and other nonmedical factors that demonstrably make a greater difference to health status than does medical progress; and, finally, an acceptance of the presently achieved average life expectancy in the developed countries as an endpoint of medical progress in its effort to overcome death—

enough now is enough. To those goals for future medical progress, I add some additional considerations pertinent to medical innovation.

1. Assume That Technology Will Increase Costs. We should take seriously a plausible assumption that, until specifically proved otherwise, almost all future technological innovations will add to the aggregate costs of health care. This has been the history of most innovations so far, and it is a reasonable assumption about those in the future; there have been no notable counter cases in sufficient quantity of late to undercut that assumption. Now, to use cost increase as a "working assumption" by no means precludes the possibility that some new innovative technologies will not increase costs or will even reduce costs; surely some will. But the burden of proof is now shifted to their proponents, who will be asked to present the evidence, or defend the plausibility of the claim, that innovation in general will help control costs.

The standard for judging technological claims should be a capacious one. It will not be enough to show that an innovation controls or reduces costs for a particular illness or episode of illness—for instance, that the rate of repeat heart attacks is reduced by a particular drug and the cost of future hospitalization is thus saved. A capacious standard will want to know (a) the additional costs of any increased morbidity from the drug treatment; (b) whether a future heart attack is *unlikely* or simply somewhat less likely; and (c) whether the likely costs of the later and final illnesses of the person saved from repeat heart attacks increase his net future lifetime health care costs.[40] The cost savings of treating a patient with drugs rather than costly operations is no savings at all if the health care costs of the life sustained turn out to be greater in the long run than they would have been if the drug had never been used. This outcome may well be a human, but not an economic, benefit—which is why it poses such a troubling ethical and policy issue.

108

2. Require That Technological Innovations Be Screened Prior to Introduction into Clinical Practice. It should be up to those who manufacture and promote technological innovations to show, in advance, that the innovation promises to be both cost-effective (economically as good as, or better than, other available alternatives) and cost-beneficial (that is, a good buy). The crucial phrase here is "in advance." Once introduced into the market, new technologies are difficult to dislodge, even if the evidence points against them. Moreover, the costs of extensive research once technologies have been introduced can be enormous. The biblical remark that "strait is the gate, and narrow is the way" should govern the introduction of new technologies.

This standard does, to be sure, present some dilemmas. It may be difficult to conduct adequate research before a technology is publicly introduced and widely adopted: a database of cases adequate to make a good judgment may not exist. It may also be difficult to put together the necessary research money if a prior evaluation is needed. The risk that an innovation will be rejected will increase, and thus so will the riskiness of the entire enterprise. Venture capital will be harder to come by.

How should these dilemmas be resolved? If the aim is a sustainable medicine, they should be resolved in favor of the standard of strictness—even if this increases the odds that the technology will not be developed. If it is true that unlimited, unfettered technological innovation is one of the sources of the high and often insupportable costs of modern medicine, and a major obstacle to sustainability, that seems the only feasible, only sensible option.

3. Establish Financial Incentives to Develop Affordable Innovations. Financial incentives of one kind or another are a powerful engine for technological innovation. In the past and right into the present, the incentives have been potently on the side of innovations, especially expensive innovations, where the profit is the greatest.[41] But those who pay for health care—whether governments, employers, insurers, or managed-care organizations—can make it perfectly clear to innovators that they are looking for ways to control the costs of technology, and that they will be unwilling to pay for expensive and economically destabilizing innovations even if these promise some benefit. At the same time, payers should encourage innovations that promise to be cost-effective, particularly preventive technologies.

This kind of message can only be delivered, I suspect, when the recipients of health care understand that rationing of care is necessary, that individual benefit cannot always be the highest standard if that benefit is excessively costly, and when the providers of care are able to use their collective purchasing muscle to gain from innovators the kinds of technologies that will be the most valuable in the long run.

4. *Invest More Money in Evidence-Based Medicine.* Though I have tried to show that technology and outcome assessment—and evidence-based medicine more generally—cannot bring about a radical control of health care costs, they can surely help. This effort will itself require a significant research investment—to improve the tools of assessment, to extend the scope of assessment, and to train those who will carry out the assessments.[42] It will no less require a wide dissemination of the results and professional and public education about how to interpret them.

5. *Indirectly Constrain Research.* There should be no direct constraints on medical research. For that matter, many forms of research need more money, particularly that basic research directed to population health, health promotion and disease prevention, and affordable innovation. But there should be the natural cooling of zeal, and investment, that would come about because of new hurdles created for the dissemination and employment of innovative technologies in the market-

place. Medical research would become a riskier economic venture; sustainability would thereby be enhanced.[43] Ample provision could be made for medical emergencies, outbreaks of infectious disease and the like. Progress would go forward, as would innovation, but more slowly, more warily, more prudently from an economic perspective. At the same time, a more systematic effort to develop research priorities could help to ensure that the innovations that do make it past the screening process would be diverted to the most important needs used in well-tested ways.[44]

The task does not end here, however. Ultimately, to achieve a sustainable medicine we must not only refashion patterns of technological innovation but look beyond the lure of technology—and the modern passion for progress—to the nature that undergirds them.

CHAPTER FOUR

Two-faced Nature:
Medical Friend
or Medical Foe?

Few tasks of human life are more demanding than the need to come to terms with nature. Nature nurtures and charms us, and nature sickens and kills us. There is "Mother Nature" and "Nature, red in tooth and claw," nature as comforting friend and nature as implacable foe. These are not two different natures, but one and the same. Medicine has throughout its history struggled to understand its relationship to mixed, troublesome, two-faced nature. One tradition, *hygeia*, has looked to the body—that most intimate product of nature—to cure and sustain itself, specifying only that it be treated with care and prudence. Another tradition, *aesculapius*, more wary and less optimistic, has looked to outside intervention, aggressive and forceful, to correct and cure the body.

Modern medicine has chosen to follow the latter path. Though gestures are increasingly made toward the "wisdom" of the body—and the possibility that a life well and sensibly lived is the best means of preventing disease—they have not had the force or glamour of a medicine that believes it must correct nature. Nature does not by any means necessarily know what is best. Just that stance, though in part correct, poses the greatest obstacle to a sustainable medicine. Yet, as I will try to show in this chapter, there can be an alternative to the spiral of medical changes, which at present always moves ahead but also simultaneously fights a rearguard action to correct the fallout hazards of earlier progress, and ever creates a more insistent thirst for continuing the forward motion. Medicine has something to learn from environmentalism about how best to understand and respond to nature. While medicine cannot defer entirely to nature, it can profitably extract some lessons from the struggle between conservationists (who work with and cultivate nature) and preservationists (who leave nature alone). The analogy I want to draw is between medicine's modern pursuit of unlimited progress and the pursuit, by global and local industry, of unlimited economic growth and affluence.

The Medical War Against Nature

"Visible nature," William James once wrote, is "all plasticity and indifference,—a moral multiverse . . . and not a moral universe. To such a harlot we owe no allegiance; with her as a whole we can establish no moral communion; and we are free in our dealing with her several parts to obey or destroy, and to follow no law but that of prudence in coming to terms with such of her particular features as will help us to our private ends."[1] The great biologist T. H. Huxley went a step further in his famous 1894 essay "Evolution and Ethics." He contended that the results of evolution are morally unacceptable and require a moral condemnation of nature. "Let us understand, once and for all," he wrote, "that the ethical progress of society depends, not on imitating the cosmic process, still less on running away from it, but in combating it."[2]

Huxley's statement could serve beautifully as a declaration of modern medicine's view of nature. Francis Bacon, the first modern figure after Descartes to chart a future course for medicine, said something similar very much earlier, when he remarked that the skills of science do not "merely exert a gentle guidance over nature's course; they have the power to conquer and subdue her."[3] Joseph Fletcher, in his 1954 book *Morals and Medicine*, brought together the theme of medicine's drive to dominate nature and the use of that domination to serve our private ends. It is choice, he believed, that gives human life its dignity, and it is the control of nature by medicine that makes the choice possible: "Just as helplessness is the bed-soil of fatalism, so control is the basis of freedom and responsibility, of moral action, of truly *human* behavior . . . technology not only changes culture, it adds to our moral stature."[4]

The medicine that emerges from this confluence of values becomes limitless in its aspirations, inherently expansionary in its internal dynamic, and subject to no serious social constraints but the "prudence" to which James would have us defer. When such a medicine is combined with an analytic and reductionistic understanding of nature, and then placed within the context of modern individualism and a market economy, it will have neither evident boundaries nor carefully considered finite goals. It is conquest without end, an unparalleled imperialism of the will and reason against the constraints of biology. The demand for prudence becomes little more than a quick look before leaping to avoid immediate dangers, not a survey of the terrain where lives altered in their destinies by medical progress will have to be lived long after the leap.

The consequences of this imperialistic view of nature have taken many decades to become clear. The triumphs and gains have been well and repeatedly celebrated. The gains cannot be denied, and they make the strongest case for the modern approach of medicine to nature. Only now coming

114

into view, however, as we have had a chance to examine the progress, is another possibility, one with more shadows and reasons to hesitate. In addition to the new problems and burdens created by the war against nature—and the backlash by nature—some hazardous ideas have been encouraged. Illness and disease have mistakenly come to be seen as biological accidents, contingent events that can be overcome. Medical progress against nature is taken not simply as a good to be pursued but as a moral imperative, as if human dignity could not exist without a relentless battle against disease and mortality. The distinction between commission, the harm directly and deliberately done by humans to each other, and omission, the failure to act against disease that might be cured, has been virtually eliminated, making medicine increasingly responsible for human fates. Those who, indifferent to the limits of nature, have called for unlimited economic growth, have often invoked the need for increased affluence and improved general well-being. They sometimes share with medicine the view that there is a moral duty to overcome nature in order that life may be improved, even if life is already reasonably good.

For medicine, the research imperative, at once an obeisance to the idea of progress and a moral demand now felt to be undeniable, draws upon this conflation of the external world and the imperious human will. There is, moreover, no perceived natural harmony between human selves and their finite bodies. The body is understood as a scene of instability, with initial harmonies soon giving away to the inevitable disharmony of disease. That is what nature gives us, and that is what must be mastered. The human body, a source of latent threat at every moment, has no intrinsic value, nothing to be protected for its own sake. In the absence of such value, there is no way to draw a moral "ought" from a biological "is." The only ought of any worth is that imposed by our moral judgment, drawn from our individual and social experience, not from our underlying biological nature, which has nothing to teach us.

115

A latter-day victim of this perspective on nature has been the life-cycle view of human life, a long-standing legacy of earlier efforts to understand the biological course of human existence. A life-cycle conception pressures us to understand human life within the context of organic life in general. A characteristic feature of that life is the rise and fall of individual organisms and the succession of one generation of organisms by another. Modern medicine, in its effort, for instance, to distinguish between getting old and getting sick, and by its response to the human dislike of aging, has all but declared the life-cycle conception an historical anachronism. Who says we have to age? That cycle can be replaced by a medicine capable at least of controlling the illness and decline associated with aging, at best of radically extending average life expectancy, and perhaps of doing both at the same time. No one claims that these possibilities are within striking distance, only that there are no theoretical scientific obstacles to such a development and only mild moral objections, easily put aside, to making the effort to bring it about. But this hope presents one more impediment to a sustainable medicine.

I would hardly want to ignore the reason why human beings resist accepting a life-cycle view. A life marked by a rise in possibilities, followed by a destructive decline—the movement from youth to old age—is surely in one respect fearful and intolerable. Who wants that? Yet at the same time, it is the fate that nature has given us. Ambivalence in the face of those two opposing realities—our repugnance at our fate warring against a perception of its power—is readily understandable. No less understandable is the tension between the now widespread desire to find ways to be less dependent on a curative, aggressive medicine to maintain health, and the fact that nature does not always, or even often enough, smile on the human body.

The Fitful Revolution

For all its force in pressing forward against nature by knowledge and technological innovation, medicine has of late witnessed a fitful revolution. This revolution—I call it fitful because it resists mainline medicine but remains willing to defer to that medicine when the chips are down—is expressed in part by the pervasiveness of the word "natural." There are "natural" childbirth, "natural" healing, "natural" food, and "natural" death, each with its enthusiastic followers. Fresh interest in traditional methods of healing is nicely symbolized and partially legitimated by the establishment, in 1992, of the Office of Alternative Medicine in the National Institutes of Health. While China may still be unusual in this respect, it has kept alive its own emphasis on traditional medicine, claiming that many of its notable successes in improving health can be traced to its merging of modern and traditional methods. Some health care systems, such as the Dutch, provide full insurance coverage for traditional as well as modern therapies. Some American HMOs are now providing alternative medicine.

The reemergence of homeopathic medicine, employing minute amounts of otherwise lethal or dangerous substances, is one more indication of the shift of public attitudes. The much-touted "holistic medicine," with its emphasis on the whole person and not just organ systems, and its embrace of natural modes of prevention and healing, is another sign of the fitful revolution. The growing attraction of medical approaches aiming to break down the standard mind-body distinction can be mentioned as well. Important here is not so much the scientific validity of these developments—evidence for them is often weak and unpersuasive—as the sheer fact of the disenchantment with mainline scientific medicine and at least a desire for something more satisfying than what it repre-

117

sents. The public hardly seems ready passively to accept René Dubos's notion that disease is a part, and a necessary part, of the total harmony of nature, but it does seem willing to adopt—however ambivalently and erratically—what might be termed a pacifist stance in the face of nature, seeking to make peace with it rather than to carry out an imperialist war of conquest.

This attraction is paralleled within medicine by the fresh emphasis on the environmental and behavioral sources of disease and illness, and by the search for nontechnological ways to reduce them. In part this development represents a rejection of the dominant, reductionist biomedical model—which seeks final genetic or organic causes of disease—and a turn to a more inclusive picture of the sources and causes of disease. But it also represents an attempt to find a less technology-dependent and biologically invasive strategy than what modern medicine has come to depend upon. Again, the pacifist note appears: if nature is understood better, it may not turn out to be so harmful after all. Nature may be at once cunning (the resurgence of infectious disease) and kinder (some people who are reasonably sensible in their living habits can live without significant illness into their eighties and nineties) than we have been led to believe. The Australian philosopher John Passmore spoke to this more complex, ambivalent attitude: "To think of nature as an 'enemy,' however, is not the alternative to thinking of it as a 'friend.' Natural processes . . . go on their own way, indifferent to human interests. But we shall do best to learn how they operate, not supposing that they will immediately respond to our whims or miraculously suspend their modes of operation so as to permit us harmlessly to convert rain forests into agricultural lands or rivers into sewers."[5] To which I would add: or to convert Alzheimer's into an improved old age, or antibiotics into a permanent resistance to infection.

The Environmental Model

It is easy enough to find some evidence of a turn away from medicine's often hostile picture of nature that has dominated the last century. Yet it is not at all evident that these signs, even when taken together, constitute a coherent and defensible alternative to the aesculapian view. They show dissatisfaction, and restlessness, and incipient revolt. But if one looks to find a well-thought-out alternative view of nature for medicine to work with, the terrain is remarkably barren. The revolt is one of feeling and sensibility, and a reaction against unhappy or excessively expensive outcomes; it is not based on a full-fledged alternative way of thinking about nature that is useful and appropriate to medicine. Can such a way be found?

The environmental movement, what I will simply term environmentalism, has thought about nature in a way strikingly different from medicine's view. In the idea of a "sustainable" environment I believe it is possible to discern a way of thinking that could be most useful to medicine.

Environmentalism as a conscious social and political movement has a long history, stretching back at least into the nineteenth century. Of course it goes back far longer, if account is taken of the many indigenous people who gave nature a high place in their culture, and of the various Romantic movements in Western culture that contrasted nature with civilization or rural with urban life. My focus here will be on the modern movement as it has animated both international and national concern for some decades now. While environmentalism as a movement is shot through with various conceptual, disciplinary, and economic disputes, four main features characterize it reasonably well. These are its stances toward nature, toward human life, toward the relationship of species in nature, and toward economic and social development.

Here are, I believe, some fair generalizations.

- Environmentalism takes a generally benign, respectful view of nature, which is seen to have a high value in and of itself. It specifically repudiates the idea that nature is an enemy, that it is infinitely plastic and resilient, or that it exists solely to serve human ends.

- Environmentalism generally stresses that human beings are only one among the full range of species that populate the earth and that the other species deserve our respect and protection. With some reservations it rejects the idea that human beings have a special, privileged place that allows them to use the rest of nature entirely as they see fit.

- Environmentalism believes that nature as a whole is an intricate and delicate web whose various parts are best understood in their relationship and interaction with each other. It rejects a piecemeal, analytical, reductionistic approach which, it believes, fails to capture the interdependence of all species. It no less rejects the optimistic idea that nature is a boundless cornucopia, resistant to any serious resource shortage that might seem to limit economic growth.

- Finally, environmentalism holds that the dominant value for economic and social development should be that of "sustainability," by which is meant the capacity of the environment to indefinitely renew itself and to maintain human, plant, and animal life in a way that will make them available to future generations.

Sustainability

The concept of "sustainability" is of fairly recent origin. The philosopher Carl Mitcham has pointed out that environmentalism has turned against the modern version of progress, which, rather than projecting an endpoint—some final heavenly city—presupposes an "indefinite and continuous superseding of the past" with no inherent limits to growth.[6] For environmentalists, limits are imperative, particularly limits on exponential growth, whether in population or food consumption, industrial production or emissions, energy consumption or land use. Environmentalists have moved from a "negative limits to growth" thesis to a more positive "sustainable development" concept.

Two important documents, *World Conservation Strategy* (1980) and the statement *Our Common Future* (1987), fleshed out this concept. Both documents take it for granted that some degree of development is necessary to satisfy human needs and to improve the quality of life, particularly for poor and developing countries that have not had the benefits of growth. But can development be conceived of in a way that takes account of the limits to exponential growth? That is the intent of the concept of "sustainable development." The biosphere must be managed in such a way "that it may yield the greatest benefit to present generations while maintaining its potential to meet the needs and aspirations of future generations."[7] At best, this is not an easy balance to achieve; for some countries, desperate to care for their people, it can seem nearly impossible.

Thus the most pressing issue behind the fashioning of the concept of "sustainable development" has been a struggle between environmentalists—concerned about pollution, the protection of natural resources, and the rights of future generations—and third-world economists and political leaders faced with severe poverty and a desperate need for economic development, even at some cost to the environment. "Sustainable development" represents a compromise between unlimited growth (the way to eventual catastrophe) and no growth, which is neither feasible nor acceptable in the face of pressing human needs. Sustainable growth is moderate, careful growth, always with an eye peeled for its immediate environmental impact as well as its long-term consequences. It is, as the term implies, development (change and progress), but sustainable (preserving the potential for meeting future needs).

Sustainability has had a special importance in the areas of energy and agriculture. With respect to energy it has been a question of conserving nonrenewable sources of energy, such as fossil fuels, while also averting the pollution and other dangers to health and the atmosphere posed by the excessive use of hazardous energy sources. With respect to agriculture it has been a matter of promoting practices less reliant on chemical fertilizers and pesticides and less likely to ruin the land for future generations. Lester Brown took the idea of sustainability a step further, introducing the idea of a "sustainable society."[8] Here the aim is not only to set limits to growth or to find ways to devise sustainable energy and agricultural policies but also to create societies that will more decisively break with modernity by embracing simpler and more frugal ways of life. By and large, however, it is sustainable development that has captured most attention, if only because of the implausibility of any quick turn to more sustainable societies.

The idea of sustainable development has not gone unchallenged. One important critique, in the agricultural area, has been that the continuing increase in food needed to meet growing populations and public demand will and must overwhelm the possibility of sustainable development. It is an idea, moreover, that more effectively serves the status quo interests of the developed countries of the West—which already have a high standard of living—than the interests of poorer countries, which are desperately trying to raise that standard. There is also in the idea of sustainability, as used by some, the belief that environmental health is simply a matter of efficiency—salvation by better management (a theme shared, as I noted in the last chapter, with efforts to develop sustainable health care systems).

As Carl Mitcham nicely sums up the environmentalist debate: "The limits to growth and the need for development are both real. The ideal of sustainable development is the name for a way that tries to recognize and bridge both realities and their sometimes conflicting claims. But the precise parameters of that bridging remain to be seen."[9] For medicine, I think it fair to say that the tension is no less pronounced: to recognize the real biological, economic, and social limits of medical progress while meeting real, still-unmet health care needs.

In the environmentalist way of thinking, no trait seems more noticeable than the interrelationship of nature and its parts. Hence, the four characteristics I earlier singled out are best thought of as a single idea with different implications and manifestations. What is that single idea? It is that human beings are an inherent part of nature and will flourish on the earth to the extent that they can understand their place in nature and successfully manage their relationship to the rest of natural life.

Two Environmental Disputes

Two disputes have been dominant in environmentalism, one philosophical, the other economic. The philosophical struggle has turned on the question of whether nature has an intrinsic value apart from human interest or human valuation. Those who believe it does have, at the extreme, held that human life is no more or less important than any other form of life; they advocate a radical egalitarianism among the earth's species. Even those who do not hold that view are, however, likely to argue that if human life is in some sense superior to other forms of life, it is still dependent upon respect for those other species and upon an effort to help them flourish, both for their own sake and for us humans who need them for our own well-being.

The other dispute is economic, though that term does not well capture the full range of issues at stake. On the one side have been the conservationists, who have held with their early

123

leader Gifford Pinchot that "the first duty of the human race is to control the earth it lives upon."[10] The quickly drawn corollary was that nature should be protected in order that it can best serve human needs, and that with wise management there is no reason it cannot indefinitely continue to do so. A sensible development of technology, a prudent husbanding of natural resources, and a careful use of market forces can both protect nature and serve human ends.

The preservationists, by contrast—with the naturalist John Muir as a central figure—have held that nature should be protected for its own sake, not for the instrumental purpose of human beings. Civilization spoils and destroys nature. Even if technology, commerce, and civilization could allow us to survive well enough, the instrumental use of nature for human goals would still be wrong. Nature has its own value apart from human life, and that value should be fully recognized, even to the point of subordinating human needs. "It is better," the environmental philosopher Mark Sagoff has noted in describing the preservationist view, "to control our wants and desires [so as] to accommodate nature . . . than to control nature to accommodate our wants and desires."[11]

It is beyond the scope of this book to pursue the details of this debate. Instead, I want to see its implications for the notion of sustainability that has come to dominate environmentalism. Both conservationists and preservationists would agree on the importance of a sustainable environment. But conservationists believe that that goal is compatible with economic and technological development; indeed, without such development a sustainable environment will not be possible. Human ingenuity, which can be benign, must compensate for the inadequacy of nature in meeting human needs, especially those of advanced developed societies. Preservationists, as might be guessed, have no such optimism. Technology and development, they hold, have created the environmental problem; simply throwing more of the same at nature will exacerbate, not relieve, the pressure. Sustainability requires a far more radical stance, the main ingredient of which is that human life must be shorn of its privileged, dominating place. It is nature that will sustain us in the long run, not human invention and intervention—but only as long as nature is allowed to have its way. While most preservationists do not often say "Nature knows best" without qualification, their ideology and practice come close to just that; some, like Barry Commoner with his "second law of ecology," say exactly that.[12]

The parallels between the environmentalist's idea of preservation and that of the medical tradition of *hygeia* are sometimes striking. As the Dutch philosopher Henk Verhoog has noted, "Both in connection with a healthy body and a healthy environment, there is a trust in the 'healing powers' of nature itself. Any interference in nature should start on the basis of this assumption. The key concept is not control but cooperation with nature. Interference combined with respect for nature."[13] The Hippocratic *Precepts* of 2,500 years ago show the ancient roots of this idea. Physicians, it enjoined, should "display the discoveries of the art [of medicine], preserving nature, not trying to alter it."[14] Verhoog calls this the "partnership" concept of sustainability.

Can Medicine Use the Environmental Model?

Two questions arise. Can the environmentalist—especially the preservationist—understanding of nature effectively be introduced into the way medicine thinks about nature? And can the environmentalist approach to sustainability be adapted to a medical context? The answers to these questions are by no means self-evident. For all its apparent congeniality with the kind of steady-state sustainable medicine I am trying to promote—and particularly its parallels with the *hygeia* tradition—I don't believe that the preservationist stance can be fruitfully adopted by medicine.

To someone steeped in the literature and practice of

medicine—full of illness, disease, and (usually) unwanted death—the environmental literature has an air of sunniness and calm. While it acknowledges that nature can destroy human life, it does not dwell on that fact. The nature celebrated by the environmentalists is usually a benign, wise, comforting reality, surely in need of care and some watchfulness on the part of humans but in all a source of life and goodness if properly respected.

The nature perceived by modern medicine, in contrast, is full of threats and harms, a nature that will eventually do us in, a nature indifferent to our individual desire to live and to have good health. Part of the success of medical screening programs—for hypertension, or high cholesterol levels, or invisible cancers—is that the public has been persuaded that the apparently healthy body can conceal a deadly, insidious nature, gradually killing us. And that is true. The nature that scientific medicine sees is amoral and often cruel. That is the nature that walks in the door of the doctor's office, or is carried into the emergency room. The nature medicine sees lacks wholeness and cohesion; above all, it displays no discernible end, in particular no end inherently congenial to human purposes. The nature that environmentalism sees is just the opposite: it gives life, it nurtures that life, and even when it brings life to an end it does so with the greater good of species and the whole as its end.

If alliances were being formed, modern medicine would be on the side of the conservationists. It would believe with them that progress is a good, and often a necessity, that nature can and must be interfered with, and that if the body as a natural object is to be respected, that respect should never interfere with any decisive act necessary to protect or advance wise human purposes. Yet there is still a difference in emphasis and tone. Modern medicine in its scientific, expansionary mode hardly pays even lip service to the value of nature or its tutelary possibilities. More commonly, it takes a briskly functional view, working to overcome or change whatever in nature op-poses its aims. What little homage there is to *hygeia* comes in a nod toward "watchful waiting" with some patients, but a waiting ready to be set aside if nature refuses to heal the body on its own. It is not a medicine tolerant of failure, and it would find odd the notion that the viruses and bacteria that harm human life have any value in their own right. The eradication of smallpox from the face of the earth was not mourned in medical circles.

Nonetheless, it should be evident by now that the modern medical view of nature has too many drawbacks to be acceptable any longer. Our medicine is beginning to run out of its capacity to dominate nature, much less dominate it in a way that is affordable. The belief of scientific medicine—like the corresponding belief of many conservationists in environmentalism—that nature is infinitely plastic and repairable, that technology can solve the problems generated by technology, that progress can move forward in a straight line, should now be seen as patently false (or, perhaps better, patently self-deceptive).

As conservationists must now know, it is enormously costly to manage industrial technology. The disposal of waste products, the preservation of clean air and water, and the avoidance of hazards to human health do not come cheap. A parallel phenomenon is no less on display as medicine pushes forward in its war against disease. Just as nuclear power plants (which produce desired energy) generate a chronic waste-disposal problem, so life extension (which produces desired survival) generates a chronic-illness problem, and on, and on, and on. Medicine ought not to adopt the kind of conservationism that sees nature as mere stuff for human manipulation, even in the name of health.

Yet if the stance that modern aesculapian medicine has taken toward nature is too radical, too little respectful of nature, neither can we go the way of preservationism. Human beings cannot survive, much less survive well, in a nature untouched by human hands, including their own human nature.

"Pristine" nature kills and sickens and cripples human life; and humans must at least take arms against it.

Some progress will always be needed, if only because human health needs and problems will change over time. *Some* manipulation of nature can improve upon nature, whether surgery for individual threats to life, or public health measures to lower infant mortality rates. *Some* wiser understanding of, and careful intervention into, nature can improve the prospects for family health, as the field of genetic counseling has shown.

For all the power of the *hygeia* tradition, it can never be enough by itself. My brief is not, then, for a medical equivalent of the preservationist position—nature untouched—but rather for a wiser embrace of conservationist ideas. The compromise position—which I will develop in later chapters—is to give *priority* (not exclusivity) to personal responsibility and *hygeia*, strengthened by public health strategies, bringing in aesculapian medicine as a secondary strategy and limiting its high-technology aspirations.

For all these reasons, then, medicine will have to find a benign equivalent of the conservationist view of nature—but with an important variant (to which I will return): a nature that kills us in painful, premature, often degrading ways can never be embraced with the kind of enthusiasm environmental preservationists, much less deep ecologists, bring to nature—which they see as innocent and nurturing, integrated and orderly. Nor can medicine, any more than environmentalism, simply choose between a preservationist and a conservationist alternative. Too little nature remains untouched by human hands, or will remain untouched, for a pristine preservationism to endure; and conservationists have come to understand the need to integrate human and nonhuman species into a coherent way of thinking about both together.

Even so, medicine can make much use of the environmentalist way of thinking about sustainability. It can use the idea that nature has value and does, if respected, have a great capacity for sustaining health and healing illness. It can use

128

the idea that a notion of sustainability too heavily dependent upon ever more technological manipulation to carry it forward is ultimately self-defeating. It can use the idea that nature is a network of interdependence and causal interactions, and thus can look at the aggregate of disease and illness and not, as now, simply isolate them from each other, supposedly the better to cure and manage them one by one.

Most important, medicine needs to adopt the environmentalist's long-term perspective, recognizing that the great imperative is sustainability over generations, not just for the next few years. The unwillingness of modern American medicine (and of the society of which it is a part) to face up to the problems of an aging population, or to the fact that infectious disease is staging a comeback, or to the implications of turning inexpensive, fatal conditions into expensive, chronic conditions shows that medicine is far from knowing either that it should take a long-range view, or what it would mean to do so.

Sustainable Nature, Sustainable Medicine

A sustainable medicine would need to understand that it cannot utterly dominate nature or manipulate it however it sees fit. The environmentalist's view of nature provides a number of helpful ways of thinking about that need, but that view must be supplemented by a recognition that human beings cannot accept—not wholly—the disease and death that come from nature. I say "not wholly" because of our understandable reluctance to passively acquiesce in our biological fate. Yet in the end—somehow—disease, death, and our biological fate must be accepted as part of our human nature. That tension between "not wholly" and "somehow" is almost unbearable, and it is hardly surprising that we will want to delay the "in the end" and to make it more tolerable.

I will formulate the full problem as follows. A sustainable medicine is one that will have to satisfy three requirements si-

129

multaneously. It will have to (1) live within the boundaries of nature, respecting and deferring to that nature and being prepared to learn from it; while (2) recognizing the human need to struggle against those aspects of nature that bring pain, illness, a loss of human functions, and a premature death; and (3) manage that struggle in some affordable way. It will then have to understand that the tension and contrary pull of (1) and (2) will have to be resolved within (3), the boundaries of a sustainable medical economy.

What are some possible strategies for meeting the three requirements of sustainable medicine?

1. *Living Within the Boundaries of Nature.* From the perspective of health and human biology, the human life cycle serves well as a foundation for living within the boundaries of nature, and as a starting point to develop a view of nature to support a sustainable medicine. All organisms have a life cycle: they come to birth, they mature, they reproduce, they flourish, and then they decline until they die. While medicine has succeeded in changing some aspects of the human life cycle, that cycle remains a fundamental of human life as of all other life. With further thought and refinement in the context of present knowledge, the life cycle can serve as the natural foundation of a sustainable medicine. It should be the aim of medicine to assist people in successfully passing through the different stages of life, from birth to maturity to old age. As I suggested earlier, there is no good reason why this cycle need be any longer, on average, than it now is in the developed nations: namely, seventy-five to eighty-two years. Let me try now to make that case more fully.

The life cycle has some key features useful in thinking about sustainability: it is limited and finite, though not rigidly fixed; it seems resistant to total domination by human agency; and it is compatible with the most common forms of organizing social and familial life, which have always had to take it into account. Its most valuable feature for a sustainable medicine is its most obvious: the life cycle has a beginning and an end, and the life of the species is that of overlapping beginnings and ends.

What would it mean to look to the life cycle as the foundation of a sustainable medicine? Why *ought* we to care at all about the life cycle, much less attempt to derive from it a moral and social foundation for sustainability? Even if we agree it is important biologically, why must that entail the practical conclusion that we should respect it? If medicine has over its long history endlessly tried to manipulate biology, why should it feel any special qualms about manipulating, or even setting aside, the life cycle if it can successfully do so? Moreover, even if we could agree that the life cycle ought to be respected, is its meaning and nature fixed or clear enough to serve effectively as a standard for medicine? Should not the increase in average life expectancy from forty-five to seventy-five years over the course of the twentieth century at least give us pause even about something so basic as its length?

I concede at once that no decisive single argument can be mounted to support the value of the life cycle as a standard. The "is" of the life cycle does not automatically generate the "ought" of it as a foundation for a sustainable medicine. Yet the case need not be made that way. Instead, we can follow what the environmental philosopher Holmes Rolston has called a tutorial way.[15] We can wonder why nature and evolution have generated life cycles in organic beings and what value that rhythm of life appears to serve. The continuation of species is one, guaranteeing a constant renewal of the vigor of species. An analogous value can be seen in human life: the coming and going of the generations creates genetic and cultural vigor in human life. Even if death comes at the end of the cycle, it has a function within the lives of individuals analogous to the role it plays within species: it forces the shaping of the narrative of a human life, which moves through marked stages each with its own possibility of distinctive flourishing.

Some of us might desire to have eternal youth, to see the

clock of the life cycle stopped at a particular point. But would this be all that good for us as individuals? There is no special reason to believe it would, and is it not easy to imagine a life perpetually stuck at one stage that would not soon come to boredom and ennui, with the possibility of significant change arrested and frozen? If life, moreover, did not turn out well at that stage, surely a possibility, the benefit would soon turn into a straitjacket. Given that prospect, time and change do not appear such terrible alternative fates.

We can gain some help in thinking through the possible place of the life cycle by taking on the question of its meaning and nature. But this can only be done by abstracting from the range and variety of individual lives within the average or general life cycle to see if we can discover and formulate an ideal form or paradigm. Here scientific progress in extending average life expectancy provides a helpful clue. While *average* life expectancy has significantly increased, this is not because most people are setting new records for long lives. There have always been some people who lived into their nineties and beyond one hundred. That is enough to show us that, under optimal conditions, some human beings can live well beyond the seventy-five to eighty-two average years now achieved in developed countries. The increase in the average has come primarily from a great drop in infant mortality rates, and secondarily from a more gradual increase in the number and proportion of those who go beyond the age of sixty-five. What we see is not an infinitely flexible life cycle but, instead, one open to considerable internal reshaping—that is, there still appear to be limits to individual life spans, with a maximum somewhere in the vicinity of 120 years. The greatest flexibility comes with the possibility of giving more and more people the possibility of avoiding a premature death and living a long old age.

Here, then, we have one positive ideal that a contemporary understanding of the life cycle makes possible. We can begin to imagine what it would be like for most people to survive youth and younger adulthood and become old people; and that imaginative act is now being achieved in reality through-out the world. We can no less imagine ways in which old age can be improved, making the time lived within the boundaries of the life cycle healthier and more functional. At the same time, however, we have now had enough experience in work-ing with an extended life cycle to know that it by no means au-tomatically produces what has been called successful aging. On the contrary, the increase in average life expectancy, and particularly the increase in the number of those older than eighty-five, has shown that nature can extract a high price for that advance: increased frailty, a greatly heightened risk of de-mentia, and a likely dependence upon others at some point in the extended life.

There are two ways we can respond at this point. We can simply see that "high price" as a scientific challenge, an obsta-cle that in principle is no different either from the high infant mortality rates that once led to shorter life expectancies, or the infectious diseases that carried earlier generations to a quicker death. Or we can see in the resistance of human biology to be-ing pressed too far into old age a piece of helpful tutoring: if you want to keep pushing at this point, after coming this far, then be prepared to pay high costs, to make only slow progress, and to achieve mixed results. You might also ask, given the economic and social costs of aged societies, whether we should push much farther in this direction at all. Medical re-search in effect wants to ignore or bypass the life cycle, which has death built into it as its natural, biologically ordained end. But if medicine is permitted to ignore the life cycle, the possi-bility of a sustainable medicine vanishes altogether.

As much as some individuals might want a greatly ex-tended life span, there is no reason a society should use its common resources to pursue that goal. The present average life expectancy in the developed countries has proved per-fectly adequate for most people to live a full life and for those countries to flourish economically and intellectually. I have heard no claims that an average life expectancy that moved from the low to the mid-eighties, much less higher, would lead to a better family life, greater economic productivity, a richer cultural and scientific life, or a generally higher standard of collective happiness and sense of well-being. While a decently long life can no doubt contribute to those goods, more life beyond a certain point seems to offer no proportionate gains. Yet I do not doubt that, even if we do not aim explicitly to extend average life expectancy, it may and probably will slowly increase. Nor can we doubt that much of the medical knowledge that will benefit the young, or help to reduce premature death, will turn out to be applicable to saving and extending the lives of the elderly; so it has been in the past and so it will be in the future. I want only to argue that policy and medical research should no longer have life extension as their aim, and that social resources should not be too readily available to individual elderly persons to pursue such a goal. Not only will there be little or no common benefit from providing such support, it is likely to increase the burden of the old on the young, a burden already now becoming a major crisis in the developed countries.

If the goal of a reflection on the life cycle is to find our way to a sustainable medicine, then we will pay attention to, and emphasize, nature's cautionary signals. Prudence would suggest that we turn our attention not to reshaping the life cycle into an open-ended set of possibilities for the species, but to improving its possibilities for individuals within the framework already provided by nature, a framework that can be perfectly adequate for human life, both collectively and individually.

I have made no argument here for deriving an "ought" from an "is," but have only suggested a way we can look at nature, allow it to say something to us, and then devise prudent and pragmatic standards to take account of some of its lessons. What we should be looking for is a plausible and helpful way of looking at nature, one that can both serve as the basis of sustainability and offer a congenial alternative to that view of nature that gives us no value, assumes there is nothing to be learned from it, and encourages us to manipulate it at will. A richer and better understanding of the life cycle offers exactly that possibility. The instigation to develop that understanding arises at just the point where nature offers strenuous resistance to manipulation and change. It is the practical, not just the theoretical, limits that should catch our eye, as the cost and difficulty of eradicating chronic and degenerative diseases should make evident.

2. *The Necessary Struggle Against Nature: Medical Progress.* What a life-cycle perspective does not so obviously offer us, however, is a way of taking account of the human need and demand not to be oppressed by that nature which sickens and kills us, and by that human nature which fervently hopes for some progress made against the most feared, deadly, and crippling conditions. But there is a way to meet this demand, and here I will once again borrow some environmentalist ideas.

Environmentalists sometimes use the term "sustainable development" to describe two requirements. One of them is an awareness that human life requires development and movement. Life is endlessly a matter of adapting to different environmental, economic, and social needs, which time and history constantly generate. The other requirement is a type of development that does not ruin the environment. Thus "sustainable development," in one helpful formulation, is understood to be "improving the quality of human life while living within the carrying capacity of supporting ecosystems."[16]

I will adapt that definition of sustainable development to the idea of medical progress in the context of a richer understanding of nature than is now common. Under a model of sustainability, medical progress should be understood as improving the quality of health within a finite life cycle in a way that seeks to avoid straining the biological or social or economic capacity of humans to adapt to the progress achieved. I mean by this definition, first, to capture the notion of a *finite* life span, thus putting out of bounds any deliberate efforts to significantly lengthen the life span of people in developed countries and, second, to signal the importance of a form of progress that incurs more aggregate and long-term benefits than burdens and that does not try excessively to circumvent the hazards of nature.

This would be, in sum, a careful and wary approach to the idea and pursuit of progress. It would look in particular at (1) the long-term consequences of the progress, and (2) the aggregate impact of progress across a number of medical fronts simultaneously. Further efforts to improve outcomes for low-birthweight babies (e.g., those weighing less than 500 grams), for example, are likely to be exceedingly expensive and to have poor long-term results; in neonatology we have reached a good place to heed the barriers nature has erected. In contrast to looking at single medical conditions and individual patients, by considering the "aggregate impact of progress" we examine how progress in one domain of medicine carries with it implications for the impact of progress in many areas at the same time, or what the progress will mean for other domains that it will indirectly influence. We have already noted, for example, the rise in death rates from cancer among the elderly, which is a consequence of a decline in death rates from heart disease, and the increase in the dementias in later old age, which is a consequence of escaping other lethal diseases in early old age. "Progress" in one area, then, means a setback in another; hence the need to look at two (or more) areas jointly.

Above all, a sustainable medicine requires an idea of progress that works within the limited framework of the life cycle, putting its efforts into eliminating diseases that reduce the quality of life within the boundaries of that cycle—and a cycle interpreted conservatively rather than in an aggressively expansionary way.

3. *Nature and Sustainable Medical Economy.* It is perfectly possible that, even if a finite life span could be accepted, and a moderate, wary approach taken to the idea of progress, re-

sources could still be strained beyond the carrying capacity of an economy. The demand then will be for a way of under-standing and managing health care that successfully deals with that strain. I will again borrow an environmental concept, that of a "steady-state economy."[17] Such an economy is the result of sustainable development, which enables the economy to maintain vigor without undue threat of resource depletion. I will thus define a sustainable medical economy as one that, having accepted the need to live within the boundaries of the life cycle, and having adopted a careful, cautious view of progress, manages to work with a steady-state allocation of re-sources to health care and to find ways to improve medicine even within that restrictive boundary. What the environmental economist Herman Daly has to say about economic systems in general could well be said of the economic system of medicine that sustainability would promote: "The three basic goals of an economic system," he writes, "must be efficient allocation, eq-uitable distribution, and sustainable scale."[18] Few developed countries have efficient health care allocation yet, though the European countries do better than the United States, just as they do with the equitable allocation of resources. The larger argument of this book, however, is that all countries are being pressured into health care systems without a sustainable scale, even if government controls and market mechanisms can de-lay the final reckoning.

I am assuming here that the nations of the world, and surely the developed countries, will not be able to devote a steadily growing proportion of their gross national product (GNP) to health care. Nor should they. That proportion will have to level off at some point; a limit will be set, politically and economically, though it may vary somewhat from country to country. Most countries are already at that limit or close to it—faced with a growing public unwillingness to pay steadily higher prices or taxes for health care, or to devote an ever larger portion of national resources to the improvement of health care. A steady-state medical economy is sooner or later

137

inevitable, and it requires a sustainable scale as its foundation. But a steady-state medical economy, if it is still to see some degree of progress and improvement, will have to find it in clever forms of technological innovation, better management, altered financial incentives—and, most of all, in public attitudes and expectations that do not press obsessively beyond what is feasible. It is too much, perhaps, to expect that any society will live easily with a steady state, either in medical progress or in resource allocation, but it is not too much to expect that, given the desire to hold down costs, the public can mute its muttering and unhappiness and adapt to the reality principle.

Yet that outcome is neither likely nor possible unless there is the beginning of an understanding that nature is not infinitely malleable, at least within acceptable costs and with acceptable medical outcomes. The next step will be to help people understand that a decent life can be had within the bounds of a life-cycle perspective on nature, and particularly its acceptance of death, and that progress within the bounds of that life cycle holds out the promise of significant gains in the future. If medicine can never adopt quite as cheery and optimistic a view of nature as some environmentalists have, it may be able to generate a way of thinking about and using nature that strikes a good balance between the hope for improved health and the limits on that hope posed both by nature and by domestic economies. One thing at least is clear: a sustainable medical economy will never be possible in the face of the still-enduring myths that medicine can forever transcend biological life and that better economic management will permit us that transcendence. Both the historical record, and common sense, should now tell us otherwise.

CHAPTER FIVE

Self, Society, and Suffering

In 1861, the great American physician and man of letters Oliver Wendell Holmes noted that "medicine, professedly founded on observation, is as sensitive to outside influences, political, religious, philosophical, imaginative, as is the barometer to the changes of atmospheric density."[1] What was true then is no less true now, despite medicine's efforts to become more scientific. The interplay of medicine, government, business, the media, and public interest is intense. Two general problems stand out in this interplay: the way medicine interacts with the individual self and its wants and demands, and the way medicine interacts with society, no less full of needs and desires. A sustainable medicine must find fruitful ways of managing those interactions. They provide its shaping context, and through them the values of progress, innovation, and the domination of nature are played out.

The idea of a sustainable medicine will have to confront three great attractions of modern medicine, which together combine and blur the line between a medicine oriented simply toward health and one that at times seems to promise a more profound human liberation. The first of these is the possibility of transforming illness and mortality, radically reducing human suffering. The promise put forward is that the causes of disease can be conquered and illness pacified; and, with illness all but eliminated, mortality itself can be transformed, the failings of a flawed and finite body brought under final control. The appeal here is both to individuals, who want to be spared the assaults of nature, and to society, eager to reduce the social burden of illness and the costs of health care. At the heart of this dual attraction is the desire to reduce suffering, that greatest of all the enemies of modernism. Suffering can come about because of social failure, as with war and crime; or through the evils done by people to each other in domestic, professional, and commercial life; or because of the ills inflicted upon us by the malfunction of our bodies. Modern medicine has aggressively challenged the ancient assumption that suffering is inherent in human life, never to be banished. It is a most popular, widely cheered challenge.

The second great attraction of modern medicine is the expansion of biological choice and medical possibilities beyond traditional limits. Here the aim is not the historical goal of avoiding disease and averting death, but of using the knowledge and skills of medicine to satisfy our personal desire for transcendence of fate: for control of procreation and a more perfect baby; for better athletic performance; for reduction in the ordinary stresses of life; for a more attractive face and body; for a happier, more relaxed personality or mood; for a more competitive height.

The third great attraction is that of helping or allowing people to live a different kind of life than was possible for their ancestors. Procreative choice, which allows women more easily to work outside the home and pursue careers, is an obvious example here. But no less striking are altered expectations about life in old age, no longer to be so burdened or crippled, and improvements in mental health that do more than simply bring people up to some level of normality. James E. Sabin and Norman Daniels, in a discussion of insurance coverage for mental health problems, helpfully distinguish among three models of "medical necessity": (1) bringing individuals up to statistical normality; (2) enhancing personal capability to allow people to cope with the world and compete in it more effectively; and, even beyond that, (3) improving individual potential for happiness.[2]

For the time being, it may be possible to hold back insurance or entitlement claims for treatment of those personal conditions that constrain the enhancement of capability or the quest for happiness. But the line is hard to maintain, constantly being nibbled at as the possibilities for drugs or therapies make those quests hardly different in practice from the older goals of simply decreasing the impact of mental disease or disability. It is equally difficult, moreover, to maintain a sharp line between benefiting individuals and benefiting society, particularly when it is argued that a principal function of society is to benefit individuals or that a society will do better with happier people. The economist's interest in the burden of illness, less high-flown in its aspirations, focuses heavily on the loss of economic productivity as a result of illness.

Even though the line between the attractions of modern medicine for individual benefit and for society is hard to discern, much less maintain in practice, I want to say more about each of them individually and then, that done, consider them together again. Mine is a dual thesis: a medicine that comes to see itself as using its skills to feed the desires of the private self, or to solve major societal problems beyond the traditional boundaries of medicine and health, cannot fail to destroy all possibility of being economically and psychologically sustainable. In the process it runs a mortal risk to its own self-identity and historical goals. Yet it is precisely because medicine can

141

increasingly offer more than the relief of disease or the fore-stalling of death that it will have a severe problem with, and face a basic dilemma about, its own mission and future. I want to press for conservative medical goals at a time when much conspires to dissolve them.

Can medicine have an internal compass strong enough to lead it to restrain its hand (a kind of negative capability), and potent enough to give it a positive direction of its own, based on some viable, sustainable notion of the human good, individual and societal? Three questions appear in the middle of the road to this goal. Which conceptions and aspirations of the modern self can medicine appropriately serve—and which must it refuse to serve? What is medicine's proper contribution to the well-being of society—and when should it resist society's aims? Hovering over both those questions is a third one, the most fundamental of all, cutting through self and society: what should medicine's role be in the relief of suffering, and which forms of suffering should it recognize as beyond its legitimate knowledge and moral scope? How each of these questions is answered will have a profound bearing, direct and indirect, on the possibility of a sustainable medicine.

Mortality, Medicine, and the Modern Self

The greatest threat to the self is that of death, the utter destruction and disappearance of the self. This is not to say that death is necessarily the worst fate that can befall the self; sometimes it is a welcome release. But that is the exception. Death in general remains an obvious threat because the possibility of life is the foundation for all other human possibilities. For pre-modern medicine, death was simply an inevitability about which it could do little; death took the lives of people across the entire life cycle. The wise doctor was one who knew, when death was on the way, to leave the scene so as to avoid any imputation that he had been its cause; besides, there were others who could be more usefully helped. Modern medicine changed all that. Where the postponing or forestalling of death had not even been a goal of an earlier medicine, it quickly jumped to the top of the list once medicine could do something about it. Where the physician could at one time offer only some comfort and palliation to the suffering, death-drawn patient, these have now become secondary goals: what one seeks to achieve when nothing else can be done.

Mortality itself soon became the enemy, approached by warfare against those diseases and conditions that cause death. In recasting its relationship to death, medicine as an institution came implicitly to think of death as an accident, a contingent event that can be at worst controlled and at best (if not quite yet) overcome.[3] Whether for the doctor at the bedside, often tortured by an anxiety that more might have been done to save the life of a patient, or for the medical researcher, full of belief that the myriad causes of death are all open to conquest, death has become remediable and avoidable, and often someone's fault: the patient's, his doctor's, his society's. "Natural death" seems now a quaint idea, and is no longer fit for death certificates. Our ordinary language has come to reflect this change. We have come to talk as if individual deaths can be averted by improved self-care, public health activities, better-trained physicians, and, ultimately, by more research. Of course death in general is still acknowledged—how could it not be?—but not necessarily the individual death of this or that patient, you or me. With enough clinical ingenuity and medical progress, that death can be avoided.

This attitude toward death—ambivalent, conflicted, working at cross purposes to itself—is at the core of modern medicine. It has the well-known result of making it difficult for physicians to deal with their dying patients; instead, they often disappear from the bedside as did their predecessors 2,500 years ago. Even worse, when death is treated as the ultimate enemy of medicine, a sustainable medicine is rendered logically impossible: no matter how successfully life is extended, or lives saved by

143

medicine, death will still be there over the next hill—different and later, perhaps, but never absent. By setting a course that challenges this reality, modern medicine sets itself an impossible biological goal, and an impossibly expensive one as well. By suggesting to an eager and equally complicit public that death can be vanquished—by the conquest, one by one, of its causes—if only adequate research funds are made available, it inevitably distorts and demeans the search for the meaning of death, which medicine cannot provide. As Dr. Sherwin Nuland has written concerning what he calls the Riddle, the drive of doctors to diagnose and then cure a patient: "To medicine's absorption with the Riddle, we owe the great clinical advances of which all patients are the beneficiaries; to medicine's absorption with the Riddle, we also owe our disappointment when we cherish expectations that doctors cannot fulfill and perhaps should not be asked to fulfill. The Riddle is the doctor's lodestone as an applied scientist; it is his albatross as a human caregiver."[4]

Modern medicine's response to death has been to say, in effect, that the problem is not to find the meaning of death but to overcome it. Death is not to be understood: it is to be *fought*. Of course, since people still die, and will always die, the self is thereby set adrift, waiting for a utopia that will never arrive while in the meantime being deprived of both motive and rationale for looking elsewhere for meaning. Fortunately, human beings are not wholly gullible when confronted by optimistic medical dreams. They turn to their religious or cultural values to find that meaning which medicine would take from them. But those values have an increasingly hard time struggling against the cultural power of medicine, which now commands a prestige few religions can equal.

Improving the Self

If death is the most conspicuous case of the medicalizing of the problems of the self, there are many other ways of doing so as well. Medicine can play to the self in two distinct ways: by normalizing it and by optimizing it. The aim of normalization, the time-honored goal of medicine, is to bring individuals up to a state of statistical normality, aiming to allow them to function in ordinary ways: to think, see, hear, and walk like everyone else. But in a medicine ever restless with its present achievements, never quite good enough in its own eyes, even this standard becomes problematic: the criteria for normality are constantly raised, keeping in step with the medical possibilities. No longer is sixty-five thought to be a reasonable age after which death is not "premature." No infant mortality rate, however low, is good enough. No ache or pain should go unrelieved if relief is desired. Most important, what would have been accepted as a decent level of health in one generation is unacceptable in the next.

Medicine can also attempt to optimize the self, playing to the individual's desire to transcend the ordinary and mundane, to go beyond the statistically normal. It can hold out the possibility of greater self-knowledge in the coming capacity to predict through genetics the probability of diseases and disabilities in the far future of a person's life. On the pharmaceutical front, the drug Prozac seems for many to have met the widespread lay desire for a drug that will improve their sense of well-being, even if they are already, by normal standards, doing perfectly well. Prozac is used by many to enhance happiness, not to cure disease or achieve psychological normality. Aldous Huxley saw this coming with his imagined soma in *Brave New World*. Prozac does for the psyche (at least, for some psyches) what cosmetic surgery tries to do for the face or the body: improve upon nature and fulfill fantasies. Prenatal diagnosis already allows couples to know the sex of their child in utero, and abortion allows them to dispose of an unwanted sex (usually female). Genetic engineering will make possible even more wish-fulfillment in the future, allowing parents to tailor the genetic traits of their offspring in ways pleasing to them. And some may want a cloned child.

145

The traditional medical goal of relieving suffering now often intermingles with the need to normalize and the desire to optimize. We can suffer because we are ill and our body has failed us. It hurts and will not function as it should. We can also suffer because either our own desires or the standards of society make us want more than we have: to be stronger, or taller, or better-looking; under less stress; more aware of our future disease possibilities. We suffer precisely because we are *merely* normal and want more than that. Medicine increasingly has the knowledge to play to that desire, and steadily it becomes acceptable for medicine to do so. The circle, to be sure, is a vicious one: the more medicine can do to improve upon normality, and thus change the standards of normality in the process, the more we will want from it. Our desires are quickly transformed into needs; and needs, we have been instructed, it is the duty of medicine to meet.

The threat all this poses to the possibility of a sustainable medicine should be evident. To render indistinct the concept of statistical normality, which ever changes as a result of medical advances, already sets the stage for a medicine that can never stand still, never reach a steady, affordable state. By playing to the desires of the self—its unwillingness to settle for less than it might be—medicine further jeopardizes sustainability. The idea of normality is soon vanquished altogether, the victim of ever-rising standards or of the pursuit of daydreams of transcendence.

None of this would be as likely, or so strong a force, if it did not play to the kind of self we have come to expect in the modern world: highly individualistic, intent on self-direction, often culturally rootless, and yet at the same time plagued by the same mortality, finitude, and limits to aspiration that marked early generations of humans. Now, however, the threatened self is often deprived of those beliefs and rituals, ordinarily religious but sometimes civic, that once allowed it to cope. The self that medicine is increasingly asked to service is a self that must, for its own survival, be ever-changing, ever on the move. It has no natural resting place save for its pursuit of desire and, with desire in hand, the escalation of desire. It is never fully satisfied with whatever is the next stage of possibility; and, in medicine, there is always a next possible stage.

The Self and the Market

If modern culture fosters the kind of self that only medical advancement can satisfy, the power of a market-oriented medicine confirms and exacerbates this drive. In response to economic pressures, as well as the spreading attraction of choice almost all health care systems are allowing—and most are encouraging—privatization and the play of market forces. Whatever its power to generate money and jobs, which is strong indeed, the market is a notably goal-less institution and set of values, practices, and attitudes. It cultivates and stimulates individual desire but has no human good or final end in mind for that desire—that is not its business. Its business is business. It wants to give people more choice about how they spend their money, and more money to spend, but it has no value system by which to judge what that money should be spent on. In fact, it promotes a way of life that aims to maximize individual preference, at the same time stimulating through the production of an unending array of goods some objects for that preference. It tells us what we might desire and prefer and how to get it, but it refuses to pass judgment on the worth of those desires and preferences. That kind of judgment contradicts its very nature, which has no "nature" in the classical sense: that of a goal built into its essence and waiting only to be expressed. Only our individual preferences, which stand beyond the judgment of the impersonal market, count.

There is the long-standing hope, to be sure, that some invisible hand will orchestrate all those preferences, those acquisitive selves, into a viable community and an affluent society. But that world is one of means only, bereft of ends. In modern medicine the market finds an ideal partner: that medicine which can cleverly and usually expensively escalate old needs and generate new desires. More important, because it can create new human possibilities, an expansive medicine is the ideal partner of the market, which must unceasingly find new products to market. And no product is so attractive as one that responds to the fear of death and the desire for health.

I do not say this as an opponent of the market in general. The market is a far more effective way to produce income and wealth than are centrally organized, state-run economies of the kind that once marked Communist or strongly socialist societies. Those simply failed, not only economically but humanly. The market is a splendid instrument for expanding the choices and possibilities open to people through medicine, and the best way of improving the economic state of a society. But there are steep prices to be paid for its contributions; and medicine is a realm in which the advantages of the market, and the human costs it carries with it, appear with a special fury.

By virtue of its drive to stimulate change, profit, growth, and expansion, the market must work to create and foster a medicine that cannot easily be sustainable, and against the kind of medicine that could be sustained. Because it seeks not only to meet old needs but also to stimulate new desires, and to transform those desires into needs, and then those needs into insistent demands, it subverts the possibility of sustainability. When the impersonal imperative of the market joins the transformative enterprise of modern medicine, the combination can only be a direct threat to the possibility of a steady-state, sustainable medicine. The same market that helps to create prosperity and to open up new horizons for people, allowing them also to pay for better medical care, can lead medicine to give up its own internal direction. In the name of health, it encourages medicine to constantly transform and transcend itself, but aimlessly. In other words, there is an intense push to improve and enhance, but with no fixed end in mind save innovation itself, with health as a rationale but actually more a slogan than a thoughtful assessment of human need.

Medicine and the Modern Self

I have laid out at some length the ecology of the modern self with which medicine must deal. It is becoming enormously difficult for medicine to retain its integrity in the face of that self's insistent demands and desires. Not only is normality subject to redefinition by medical advances—which makes it difficult to use normality as a standard for maintaining medicine's integrity—but medicine's knowledge and skills can be put to nonmedical uses, many but not all of them benign. The market simply intensifies and organizes tendencies already present.

Which conceptions of the self ought medicine to serve, and which should it refuse to serve? The answer to this question cannot be found wholly within the traditions of medicine, which have changed over the centuries in any case, and which have never before had the capacity to change the self. The fact that medical progress—whether through technology or simply improved public health—forces changes in the concept of normality tends to make that concept less and less useful to help medicine draw its own line when confronted with external pressures. Medicine, in short, seems poorly situated to cope well with the demands of the modern self.

Nonetheless, some rough standards can be suggested, which will need much further elaboration. First, insofar as it can do so, medicine should refuse to use its skills in the service of those who aim to transcend or enhance normality. Medicine is poorly placed to know what would count an improved state of human life. It can genuinely plead agnosticism on that point and refuse to serve. The fact that some human beings want to transcend some trait or condition is not sufficient evidence of the value of doing so. Second, in answering the question of whether a given desire for enhancement should be met, only a showing of demonstrable benefit should be decisive; it should not be sufficient merely to show an absence of visible harm, either to self or others. The nature and long-term value of the benefit need justification. Medicine does not, however, possess the kind of knowledge needed to determine what would count as an enhancement benefit.

Now, my first two standards would seem to close the door to any medical cooperation with that modern self that seeks to transcend ordinary biology. Yet that conclusion is probably too strict, too narrow, and surely likely to be pushed aside. Hence, it is necessary to add that medicine *may* (not "must") serve the desires and needs of the modern self when there is some clear and well-settled democratic consensus that it ought to do so. It should not be sufficient, then, that some individuals want for their selfhood what medical skills can give them; this desire must be subject to public debate and politically ratified. The principle here is that what medicine can do for individuals will almost certainly have social consequences, and thus requires community approval.

Self, Society, and Medicine

I have tried to specify some conditions that might protect medicine's integrity and the society it would serve. Fortunately, there is more to this tale than I have so far related. If the modern self, that individualistic self of open-ended, aimless plasticity, were married only to the market, there would be no hope for a sustainable medicine. Sustainability would be literally unthinkable for the inhabitants of a world given over to those values. Medicine could only go forward, growing and expanding, stopped not by its internal integrity but only by brute economic scarcity. We might then get a medicine that, even if stopped, would still be both imprudent (because it stopped at too high a level of resource consumption) and humanly poor, grounded only in clamorous wants, not in any politically, morally, or socially justifiable way of life.

The crucial variable here is the nature of the society in which modern medicine is situated. For, as with the market generally, it is society—social mores, predilections, values, and cultural institutions—that will affect the tastes and preferences of individuals, that will encourage or discourage different possible manifestations of medicine, and that will work out the nature of the tacit social contract between medicine and the market. A very general question might be asked at this point: how can society best help medicine to be the kind of institution that will be most beneficial to society and those individuals who make it up?

I think it helpful, however, to ask two additional questions to more carefully specify the issues at stake. Each is the mirror image of the other, and each is designed to help us think about what is at stake in the way medicine interacts with society, and the way that interaction works its way back into the self of those who, at once, live within society and, when sick, live within the arms of the institution of medicine. The two questions I would pose are these: What kind of medicine is best for society? What kind of society is best for medicine?

I ask these questions with some assumptions in mind, which it would be well to set forth. The most central of them is that medicine has become so important a social institution that its values and results will affect, and change, society. At the same time, the values of modern society are so strong and so pervasive that they will influence, and change, medicine. Modern society and modern medicine, then, will mutually work upon and affect each other; they can only with difficulty be distinguished in the way that happens, so subtle yet so pervasive is their interaction.

What Kind of Society Is Best for Medicine?

To ask "What kind of society is best for medicine?" is already to understand that medicine cannot be fully protected from the demands made upon it from the outside, and that it will take on, to a greater or lesser extent, the coloring of the society in which it exists. Nonetheless, if the issue to be pursued is that of encouraging and nourishing the idea of a sustainable medicine, it is possible to imagine some standards that a society could honor and could work to make effective. By "society," I mean here the cultural, educational, legal, and political institutions and practices that bind a people within a nation into an integral community.

Above all, society should allow medicine to seek its own internal goods and integrity, recognizing that a weakening or breakdown of that integrity will hurt both medicine and society. In this sense, society must be protective of medicine, working to reinforce its values and honor its practitioners. It should no less work to foster in medicine the best (if not always honored) parts of its own traditions: truth-telling, compassion, respect for individual dignity and rights, the encouraging of professional ethics and behavior, and the sheltering safeguards of the law.

By invoking this role for society, I am already implying a feature of the good society: its respect for the values and integrity of the institutions that constitute it. It does not usurp their power or rightful autonomy. It encourages their flourishing, reinforces the virtues they espouse, and intervenes only when necessary to prevent harm.

Medicine is one of those institutions. But it should not be expected to do the work best left to other institutions. It cannot be expected to relieve all suffering, or to solve the problems of poverty or violence or the breakdown of the family. As the terrible experience of Nazism shows, a medicine that becomes

152

the handmaiden of the political order is a medicine that has itself contracted a fatal illness, that of turning its healing skills into the skills of the torturer and the killer. And while medicine and the health care system can and must make some use of the market and market concepts, they ought not to be treated as just one more economic institution to serve the financial welfare of society. The fact that a health care system can be a source of jobs, that medicine can create affluence on occasion, is no reason whatever to twist them deliberately to serve those ends. A good society would take care to protect medicine from economic misuse. A good society would no less refuse to make use of medicine to help manage its life and problems. Social engineering in general, whether economic or genetic, is not a proper role for medicine, and a society is wrong to look to medicine as a vehicle for its own purposes. However valid those may be, it is invalid to see in medicine a way of achieving them.

In sum, that kind of society is good for medicine which allows medicine to serve the purposes of health, not the many other purposes that a society must serve. It is precisely here that the distinction must be made between medicine as an integrated institution with its own values and traditions, and medicine as simply an assemblage of discrete knowledge and skills. Society—whether in the form of government, or commerce, or political management—will always be tempted to draw upon those skills for its ulterior purposes. A good society is one that recognizes this temptation but learns how to resist it. Of course it is not "society" as a whole that acts, but its legislators, public officials, and moral guides.

There is a final, and critical element of the good society that must come into play. A society that is good for medicine will be animated by ideals of solidarity. Medicine's primary goal is to minister to the pain, suffering, and threat of death that the body inflicts upon us when it goes awry, when it withers, when it fails altogether. Medicine can, and will, see and treat us as individuals, living alone and privately with our finitude and mortality. But medicine will also see us collectively, as individuals with a common fate, and will recognize that its mission is social and not just individual. The company of doctors and health care workers is joined to the company of the sick and the soon-to-be-sick in a common enterprise. A society marked by a larger sense of solidarity, where each person accepts a duty to bear some responsibility for his neighbor—in education, in the creation of jobs, and in resistance to crime and incivility and the ruinous clash of racial or religious or ethnic groups—will be better able to foster and support the help each of us needs when ill or disabled. Solidarity against the evils of sickness should ideally rest upon a broader solidarity that aims at mutual flourishing and shared security.

What Kind of Medicine Is Best for Society?

Yet medicine cannot let itself become utterly dependent upon the goodwill of society, nor can it always be assured of a supportive social solidarity. Its only real protection is its internal principles, virtues, and values, potent enough to keep society at bay and to keep its own members on the right track. The great temptation of modern medicine will be to court the favor of society, and to flatter itself by offering ways to medicalize society's problems, to put itself in the service of society beyond the protection of health, and to take unto itself roles that society would gladly unload on other institutions if it could.

When it would medicalize aging, or social psychopathology, or childhood, or education, medicine fails its own mission, putting its skills out for social hire. Medicine should not—through psychotherapy or drugs or techniques of behavior modification—offer to find a shortcut through the enduring religious and philosophical questions that must afflict human beings. It can help relieve some of the physical symptoms that the enduring of such problems can generate, and some of the psychological manifestations as well. That is appropriate, but very different from medicine's offering itself as a substitute for other forms of knowledge and insight and behavioral change.

Nor should medicine come to believe that its good is equivalent to the good of society. There may on occasion be direct conflicts between its needs and those of other institutions: health may have to compete with education for resources, and roads must be built as well as hospitals. Medicine should, then, understand health to be a fundamental human good, but not the only such good or at all times the highest good. A medicine of the kind that has developed in the United States, where 14 percent of the gross national product is devoted to health care, is one that has lost its own sense of proportion. It has, instead, adopted the sensibility of a society that has allowed health care needs and claims (inefficiently and expensively delivered) to go almost unchecked and unjudged. Medicine itself cannot remain neutral about its own place in society or, like economics, work independently of goals and purposes. It ought not to be a discipline and profession of means only.

In the end, medicine will not be able to be the kind of institution that will be good for society unless it has its own internal, self-directing goals and principles. It needs them for protection against the demands that will be made upon its socially exploitable skills. But it needs them no less to chart its own course. It must have its own vision of individual and societal good, one that will animate its work while at the same time helping to shield it from inappropriate or wrongful uses. This is a minimal condition of a medicine worthy of respect— and, as I will try to show, also a minimal condition for a sustainable medicine. A medicine that is not in control of its own life, that has allowed itself to become the servant of society, even in the name of goods and goals worthy enough in their own right, is in no position to become sustainable.

Models of Medicine

In thinking about its relationship to society, medicine can use several scientific and social models to determine the nature and direction of its research and clinical application. If medicine needs to resist some demands made upon it by society, that does not mean that it should overlook, in pursuit of its legitimate medical mission, the social and economic determinants of illness and disease.

Two broadly competing models have emerged, the biomedical and the biopsychosocial–health field model. The first, historically most dominant, looks to a reductionistic and analytical science to provide the ultimate answer to human disease. The reigning model of the body is that of a complex machine, and the task of the doctor is to correct its breakdowns and defects. Medical research, as if it were peeling an onion, seeks to move from the biological and physiological levels down to the cellular and molecular levels, biology finally giving way to chemistry and physics. The aim is a full and comprehensive understanding of disease reduced finally to its core and causal elements. With that knowledge in hand, medicine looks to the ensuing possibility of a definitive cure, not simply a halfway technological repair job.

Much of the current excitement about molecular genetics, thought capable of finding the ultimate causes of disease, reflects the power of the biomedical model: go deeper and deeper and look for a single final key. Disease itself, in this model, is understood to be a deviation from a statistically measurable biological norm caused by some destructive physiological change. That change is itself caused by an excess or deficit of some critical factor, by some unknown harmful agent. A successful medical intervention requires a counterattack against that agent, neutralizing its force or compensating for its deficiencies.[5] This intervention can be seen either as an effort to discover a specific cause for a specific disease or to find the agent that harms the overall systemic balance of the organism. Disease is, in any case, not a human construct but an independent, biologically measurable deviation from a norm.

Health, in this model, is understood narrowly as the absence of disease. That absence can objectively be determined by deviations from species-typical bodily functioning. A healthy person is someone whose organs function well and who can effectively cope with the environment in which she lives. Health is thus meant to be a value-free concept.[6] A person who cannot work, a typical species function, is unhealthy; and a pancreas that should produce a sufficient supply of insulin but fails to do so is diseased. With this understanding of health in place, other concepts fall into line. Illness is to be understood as the individual's perception that he or she is suffering from a disease, a perception rooted in the observation that some ordinary level of function is absent (paralysis) or deranged (fever). Sickness is then seen as the social category into which people are placed when they are ill and which allows them various social privileges and exemptions. If you are sick, you are excused from work and also deserve the sympathy of others.

What I have been describing might best be thought of as the mainline clinical understanding of medicine. It looks to discovery of the essence of disease, moving first from the ill patient (who reports her experience of illness to a doctor), then to the doctor (who tries to find the underlying disease that is causing the illness), and then to the research scientist (who tries to find the underlying mechanism causing the disease). Only scientific medicine, not society, can determine what is truly a disease and what can be done about it. As for technology, this model of medicine welcomes it as an enormous benefit to patient welfare and a way of using scientific knowledge for clinical ends.

In recent years there has been widespread dissatisfaction with the biomedical model. That reaction has generated a number of efforts to develop a more nuanced model of medicine. While it seeks to maintain to some degree its foundation in the clinical traditions of scientific medicine—that is, it does not altogether reject reductionism—the alternative model wants at the same time to set disease and illness within a much broader causal network, linking the inner biology of people to their external social setting. The physician George Engel has been the most articulate and sophisticated proponent of what he has called a biopsychosocial perspective.[7]

The most prominent note of the biopsychosocial model is its rejection of the reductionist, wholly science-based, biomedical understanding of human health and illness. This rejection moves in two directions. At the clinical level, the rejection is based on the perception that there is no necessary correlation between illness and disease, and that in any case it is illness and its effects on their lives—not simply organic symptoms and maladies—that patients present to physicians. Two particular subjects of criticism are (1) the failure of the scientific model, biased toward cure, to offer an incentive for the care of patients with chronic diseases; and (2) the model's indifference to the suffering person as distinguished from the diseased organ.

In research, the rejection of the biomedical model is based on a variety of insights, some of them scientific, others social and humanistic. These include the now commonplace observations that (1) many diseases have ultimately environmental and social, not biologically pathological, causes; that (2) biological pathogens do not, in any event, express themselves the same way in all organisms—which is to say that there are enormous differences in individual responses to disease; and that (3) efforts to reduce biology to chemistry and physics utterly ignore the obvious complexity of human life, a complexity that deserves richer and more subtle research paradigms. For George Engel, reflecting on his own clinical experience, "It is through dialogue that the physician learns the nature and history of the patient's experience and clarifies on the one hand what they mean for the patient, and on the other, what they might mean in terms of other systems of the

158

natural hierarchy, be they biochemical and physiological, or psychological and social."[8]

This is what the educator-physician Dr. Kerr White characterizes as good clinical reasoning, which requires knowing that patient as a person and the biochemistry of the patient as well. The Canadian economist Robert G. Evans has performed a parallel task in his efforts (along with others) to understand — using a "health field" framework — the determinants of health in the individual.[9] These turn out to be a combination of social and physical environment, genetic endowment, and a variable individual response to biological threats. Just as good clinical medicine in pursuit of individual health ought not to be reduced to a biomedical approach, neither can individual health be understood apart from a web of social and environmental relationships.

Pluralism, Medicine, and the Human Good

Yet we come here to a difficult and disturbing dilemma. Medicine can and should have its own picture of the appropriate scientific model, and I believe the biopsychosocial approach is the most promising. But in developing such a model, medicine remains in its own domain. Can or must medicine move out of its scientific world, however, to have its own vision of individual and societal good? If it does not have its own vision, then it is likely to have one foisted on it, or simply to be insinuated into it. Medicine will be up for grabs by those with the most power or social influence. Yet how can medicine be expected to have its own vision of the human good if, of its nature, it is only one of many social institutions and, moreover, one that has no special access to a view of the human good? There is no easy way out of this dilemma, but I want to suggest a direction that might prove helpful here.

Three questions must be asked at this point. One of them is whether in medicine's practices, historical values, and traditions, a coherent picture of the human good can be discerned. Or has medicine for so long been influenced by, even now and then infected by, external values to such an extent that there is no picture of the human good that can be attributed solely to the internal life and characteristic practices of medicine? Moreover, even if medicine *has* worked with some discernible idea of human nature and need in mind, some idea of the individual good, is that in itself any reason why it should stay within that framework in the future? These are all questions concerning the nature and goals of medicine.

No less important is the struggle between liberal and communitarian ideologies of the self and society. Liberalism as a political philosophy has characteristically focused on individual rights, self-determination, and a notion of the self that transcends cultural rootedness.[10] In the belief that the right trumps the good, liberalism displays its skepticism of the idea that there can or should be a commonly accepted and substantively rich view of the human good, individual or social.[11] Communitarianism, by contrast, puts the common good first, noting that all individuals are necessarily also social creatures. It holds to the belief that a deep though not necessarily full realization of the human good can be perceived and embodied in the laws, customs, and institutions of society. A society is not just a minimal framework of laws and procedures to keep the peace but a joining together of people to seek some common good and common meaning.[12]

The story of the long struggle between liberalism and communitarianism need not detain us here, nor will I discuss recent efforts to find in liberalism a stronger communal foundation than is granted by its critics. What matters for my purpose is the crucial difference made by medicine's alliance with one or the other ideology or some combination of them. The quasi-market and individualistic orientation of American medicine at one pole, and the communitarian bent of European welfare-state, universal-health-care medicine at the other pole illustrate well the implications of these ideological alliances.

160

The result is not simply a different view of the obligation of government to provide health care, but a different way of thinking about the place of medicine in human affairs more generally. The contrast between the American emphasis on choice and freedom as the most important moral values for a health care system, and the European emphasis on communal solidarity is thus only one index of the difference ideological alliances make. No less important is the way that medicine itself comes to be understood.

A traditionalist medicine, oriented toward the maintenance of health (understood as species-typical functioning), allied with a communitarian political ideology, will be a medicine wary of moving outside long-standing boundaries. It will have an understanding of the human good that requires medicine to care for the health of the body and the mind, the foundation of other human capacities. But it will not look to satisfy all private desires or optimize the human condition. In contrast, a modernistic medicine, oriented toward putting the knowledge and skills of medicine to whatever ends please people so long as no flagrant harm is done, and allied with a liberal, individualistic ideology, will not hesitate to set most boundaries aside. When that alliance is sweetened by a marriage with the market, there will be economic as well as human incentives to positively rush past traditional barriers; the creation of new medical desires and medically inspired ways of life will become natural and imperative.

The implications of these alliances for a sustainable medicine quickly become evident. The combination of a modernistic medicine and a liberal political ideology means that neither medicine itself nor the larger social ideology within which it exists have any intrinsic goals or any sustained view of the human good. There is thus no social foundation, except gross economic scarcity, for a sustainable medicine. A traditionalist medicine combined with a communitarian ideology does, however, offer the possibility of a sustainable medicine: it is constrained both from within and from without.

161

The experience of the European countries since the end of World War II provides the best laboratory for testing this thesis, and indeed has inspired me to advance it. Those countries have provided universal health care while managing until recently to control costs. The core sustaining value for that universality has been solidarity, not an individual right to health care (though some countries use rights language also). It was taken for granted that, if universal care is to be made available, it can only be done by limiting and controlling technology, salaries, and fees; by some form or other of global budgeting; by a strong guidance from government; and by minimizing the impact of market forces on the delivery of health care. Rationing was understood to be the necessary corollary of universality. Europeans had, at least through the early 1990s, a sustainable medicine: equitable, economically affordable, satisfactory to and even popular with citizens, and thus psychologically sustainable. European health care systems threatened neither the quality of health care nor other societal needs. Just the opposite situation has marked the United States: we see widespread public discontent, ever-rising costs, and the diversion of resources needed elsewhere to feed a health care system at once fragmented and inefficient.

European sustainability was not simply a function of the types of health care systems found there. Background cultural values helped to make those systems work. There was less obsession with medical progress and technological innovation, less perfectionism and risk avoidance, a greater acceptance of mortality, a less hostile stance toward flawed human nature, a greater willingness to accept some degree of pain and suffering as normal, not necessarily a medical target, and less public demand for the latest and best. For the most part, European medicine was traditionalist, more paternalistic, less interested in the use of medicine to enhance life, and more fatalistic than ours. But that perhaps fortuitous combination produced a sustainable and, for a long time, a steady-state medicine.

Some Nagging Questions

At this point, however, some skepticism and a dose of reality are in order. Three nagging queries emerge to challenge the way I have developed my analysis. First, can it really be said that what I have called traditionalist medicine has as tidy a picture of its goals—of preserving or restoring a given level of normality—as I have suggested? Second, is the combination of a traditionalist medicine and a communitarian ideology likely to be possible in the future? Third, can some plausible middle ground be devised in the years ahead between an unfettered modernistic, liberal, market-driven medicine admitting no boundaries, on the one hand, and a traditionalist, limited, communitarian medicine, on the other?[13]

As to the goals of a traditionalist medicine, it is possible to trace over the centuries some enduring themes and ends. From the perspective of the doctor-patient relationship, medicine has always and everywhere taken the sick and suffering patient as its point of departure. It is the patient who confronts the doctor and calls upon his or her skills to find relief. From the perspective of culture and political arrangements, however, a far more varied scene reveals itself. There we see a plurality of meanings attached to illness and disease, a variety of conceptions of the role of the doctor, and of course a wide range of political and economic arrangements for the provision of medical care. This variety in turn shapes the doctor-patient encounter in different ways and has allowed a rich variety of meanings and relationships.

In the post–World War II West, the doctor-patient relationship has remained central. But it has been radically influenced by technological developments, complex financing arrangements, and the inroads of the surrounding culture. Those phenomena have been able to determine the interior life of medicine far more than was possible when medicine was a simpler, more insulated, and less expensive enterprise. There is nothing in the previous history of medicine to suggest some monolithic historical reality. Variety has always marked the manifestations of medical goals. The more extensive interaction of medicine and society we see now and almost certainly will see in the future means that medicine will have to struggle much more to maintain its own direction and integrity. But it cannot do this without having some hard core of conviction about its own mission, and some view of the human good with which to work.

As for the second query, it will be harder, not easier, in the future to sustain a traditionalist, communitarian medicine. Recent trends in European health care show why: costs have become difficult to control and every country is beginning to have some degree of health care strain and even crisis. The demands of the European public are increasing, not decreasing, and in particular are challenging the paternalism that has been a mark of the traditionalist-communitarian arrangements; doctors can no longer so easily keep information from patients or make all decisions for them. In order to better manage both rising cost and rising public demands, parts of the European national health care systems are rapidly being privatized, and with that movement comes heavy reliance on market strategies, concepts, and ideology.

Thus, the very ingredients that have in the past made a sustainable medicine possible in Europe—the moral value of solidarity and a government domination of the provision of health care—are beginning to show signs of stress. So far, however, that stress has not reached a breaking point; the European commitment to universal health care remains intact. The future will depend on whether efforts to control costs, and the escape valves provided by some degree of privatization, are successful. If the ultimate triumph of the market is to be avoided, however, the value of solidarity must remain strong, even if adapted to contemporary values and economic pressures. The political scientist Deborah Stone contends that solidarity is still strong among the European public, though not necessarily the policy elite; if so, the stage is set for future conflict.[14] Short of a nasty, brutish commodification of medicine, an affirmation of solidarity is the only way to maintain a humane sustainability.[15]

Solidarity is possible only when two conditions are met. First, there must be a public willingness to share the burdens of health care costs and provision; second, the tax demands made upon the public to do so must not be excessive. During the 1970s and 1980s, stability was achieved in both respects. But by the early 1990s that stability began to crack as health care costs increased. Something had to be done, and that something was a renewed effort at cost control and an opening up to the market. Because of stagnant economies, high unemployment, and public resistance to higher taxes, the option of increasing taxes to keep pace with rising health care costs was ruled out. In the United States resistance to higher taxes and to a larger government role led to the failure of the 1994 reform effort, throwing the country into an embrace of managed care and producing continued growth in the number of uninsured people. If the European countries found their commitment to solidarity reaching some limits, the United States found that it could not effectively move toward solidarity at all.

Suffering, the Self, and Solidarity

Can the civic and moral resources be found to sustain solidarity in Europe and to give it a chance of future life in the United States? Much will depend, I believe, on the response to a problem that is rarely mentioned in the political and economic debates on health care: that of the appropriate response to the suffering caused by poor health and the threat of death.

At the core of medicine lies an effort to respond to suffering that reflects John Stuart Mill's faith that "All the grand sources . . . of human suffering are in a great degree, many of them almost entirely, conquerable by human care and effort."[16] But what kind of suffering can medicine respond to? Human beings can suffer from many causes: economic deprivation and poverty, war and civil unrest, thwarted love and the destruction of relationships, grief and despair, meaninglessness and anomie. Suffering's forms are many, their causes myriad. One or all of those forms and causes may present themselves to the doctor, for just about every form of suffering can have a physical and psychological manifestation. Despair can produce depression; threatened love can bring on anxiety; war and poverty can maim and kill. But medicine cannot be expected to stop war, reduce poverty, save troubled marriages and ruined romances, or give meaning to a universe that may, to some, seem cold and indifferent to human fate. Which kinds of suffering, then, are legitimately in medicine's domain and which are not?

Medicine can legitimately deal with physical pain. Bodies can hurt, and medicine has the skills to limit or eliminate pain. It can also, through psychiatry and psychology, help people cope with suffering—that is, the experience of misery, or a threat to the self, or the anguish of chronic pain. What medicine cannot do is explain why humans are subject to pain and suffering (apart from physical and psychological causes), what those experiences mean in the larger scheme of things or in the lives of individual people. Nor can it claim to know just which forms of pain and suffering are morally acceptable and which are not—that is a matter for conscience and moral judgment, neither of which can reasonably spring from medical knowledge, which is of necessity limited and partial.

An objection might arise here. Is not medicine concerned with the whole person, and does not a biopsychosocial model of medicine imply, even require, an embrace of the full scope of human suffering? Not at all. To say medicine should encompass the whole person does not mean that medicine can or should be master of everything that concerns people. Human knowledge, for one thing, goes well beyond medical knowledge, and its impact on a person's self-conception and action may have nothing to do with medicine. Knowledge and appreciation of the arts, on the one hand, and of history, on the other, provide two obvious examples of that truth. There are, at the same time, ways of thinking about life and human meaning outside of medicine—for instance, literature, philosophy, and religion. To say, then, that medicine should focus on the whole person, a sensible enough view, must mean that it can take on the whole person only with the knowledge and skills at its command, which are valuable but limited.

Now, it is true that medicine can respond to the bodily or psychological symptoms of fears, anxieties, or despair provoked by other spheres of life. Medicine can obliterate physical pain with morphine, reduce anxiety and despair with psychotropic drugs, and restore appearance with cosmetic surgery. But there will always remain the problem of when these interventions are justifiable, and the answer must come from moral judgment outside of medicine. Medicine ought not to wipe out all grief, or dull sensibility to all tragedy, or render people stupidly content. It then trespasses into territory beyond its scope, threatening its own legitimacy as well as that of other human domains.

Suffering has two aspects. One of them is our own suffering, whether in the actuality of sickness and certain death or in our anxiety about them. The other is the way we respond to the suffering of others. While our own suffering, or the imagination of our possible suffering, can generate empathy for the suffering of others, that is by no means inevitable. We may be so absorbed in our own fate that the fate of others is pushed out of our mind, or never given a chance to enter. We can desire to help others, to relieve their suffering, but simply find ourselves unable to do so for lack of emotional or financial resources. We can also embrace political and economic ideologies that allow us to evade calls upon us to do something directly about the suffering of others. We may have empathy for the suffering of others but expect government or the market or simply their own personal efforts to take care of it.

In response to this range of possibilities, I want to suggest that how people think about their own suffering, and then relate that suffering to the similar fate of others, is likely to determine the prospects of solidarity as an animating ideal in the years ahead. Two points need to be made. The first is that an excessive individual fear of suffering combined with a perfectionistic drive to utterly abolish it will almost certainly guarantee the death of solidarity. The second point is that a viable idea of solidarity requires an acceptance of limits to health care imposed upon all and, accordingly, a reining in of personal and individual demands for health care. For a time, precisely this situation prevailed in Europe and Canada, and only in the 1990s did it begin to crack.

The Self and Suffering

One way to characterize the institution of medicine is to say that is has an integrated way of coping with the pain and suffering caused by disease and illness. Medicine's point of departure is the report of a patient that she is ill, that something is awry with the body or mind, and that mild or severe distress is present. The illness in itself is rarely the problem. It is the suffering the illness is likely to cause, or is already causing, that motivates the patient to do something. What is the response to this moment, what motivates the patient to do something about it, and what are the range of options sought by the patient?

These are crucial questions for the future of a sustainable medicine. The way the patient responds to illness will, in great part, be a function of the patient's values, the expected response of the society in which the patient lives, and the skills and resources available to respond to the needs, desires, or demands of the patient. It is evident that the patient can respond in a number of possible ways. The patient may, stoically, simply decide to bear the pain or suffering without seeking help or expecting any societal response; at best, the patient may seek not medical help but only the comforting presence of other people. The malady that afflicts her may be interpreted as just life itself, to be borne as well as one can, with personal courage and endurance. Indeed, the person who responds this way remains just a suffering person, not becoming a patient at all, which implies putting oneself in the hands of medicine. For the most part, a stoic response will be elicited either because the particular kind of suffering is not socially understood to be open to a medical response, or because even if it is, the individual decides not to avail herself of it. While this refusal of, or indifference to, medical care is rare, it is not absent and may be growing more common.

Alternatively, and far more commonly, the suffering person can decide to call upon the health care system for relief. This will ordinarily happen because society has tutored people to understand that certain forms of suffering call for a medical response, and that such a response is available to them. At this point, expectations become critical. A patient may, at one extreme, expect a medical response, but not much of one. Her expectations may be modest and undemanding, marked more by hope of help than insistence upon relief. Medicine is not expected to provide unfailing success, much less miracles. This is more or less the kind of expectation that Europeans had of their medicine and health care systems from the 1940s through the 1980s. While medical help is wanted, it is understood that all life brings some suffering, that suffering must be borne, and that medicine cannot be expected to relieve all of it.

At the other extreme of patient expectations is what might be called the insistent modern response. A person suffers from a real or suspected malady. He then expects medicine to provide full relief from that condition. The demands upon doctors are high, and failure to deliver relief is not readily accepted. Suffering is not to be tolerated. If a treatment fails, it is probably someone's fault, possibly a malpractice case, not the result of an inherent limitation in medical knowledge or skill. And should there turn out to be such a limitation, it is imperative that research direct attention to overcoming it, to finding a cure. It becomes the duty of society to support the research that will reduce suffering. Suffering is not to be accepted or understood, but only to be erased. Medicine has too often been caught up in the liberal ideology that, in the words of the theologian Courtney Campbell, "There exists a direct and necessary connection between the preservation of human dignity (i.e., choice and control over the powers of life and death), and the absence of suffering and dependency."[17]

This kind of response naturally feeds medical perfectionism and a steady lowering of the threshold of what counts as intolerable suffering. No complaint is too minor to be considered fodder for a research assault, and no degree of medical risk too inconsequential to ignore. This kind of response also fuels public demand for presymptomatic screening and for the advancement of predictive medicine. The transformation of suffering—historically a problem of life itself—into simply one more medical challenge has two profound effects: it helps to create an unsustainable medicine and, at the same time, dampens efforts to find philosophical or religious meaning in suffering. The latter consequence is just as harmful as the former. Meaning has always been difficult to find, but when the search itself is denied as meaningful—when it is transformed into an effort to rid life of suffering altogether—the consequences are all the more debilitating. That denial promotes a brand of medical narcissism, turning people in on themselves as they search for medical relief, and it promotes an insatiability in that narcissism, leading people on to ever more insistent and higher demands to have their suffering relieved. Nothing is ever quite good enough, particularly a human body that refuses to behave perfectly. As it will.

Suffering and Solidarity

It is no accident that the idea of a right to health care and the idea of solidarity as the foundation for health care have together come upon hard times. It soon became evident, in the American context, that the language of rights was open to unlimited claims, with no obvious way within the context of rights to set limits to them. When a rights perspective is combined with insistence on equal, universal access to health care, the possibility of excessive demands is patent. When to this mix is further added the belief that a right to health care is tantamount to a right to the relief of suffering—and suffering perfectionistically understood—the entire venture becomes insupportable. When a right to health care becomes a right to be relieved of the suffering of life, it has no future. It makes no sense in its own terms, nor can it financially be supported.

While solidarity has fared comparatively better within the European context, it has suffered somewhat from the virus that has afflicted the American scene. The demand for improved health care, for wider coverage of a wider range of conditions, has forced up the cost of care. Worse still, the narcissism that goes with the unlimited quest for perfect health affects not only attitudes toward disease and illness but also the sense of obligation to others. Nothing seems more offensive to an individualistic and market-oriented medicine than a contention that limits must be set on the provision of efficacious medicine. Individual benefit is thought to be the only acceptable standard for providing health care—not age, or cost, or the needs of particular groups.

But the key to European solidarity has been the mutual willingness of people to live with limits in order that everyone can have, if not *perfect* medicine and health care, *decently adequate* medicine and health care. Solidarity, in short, requires some degree of self-sacrifice. But if self-sacrifice itself is seen as

171

a kind of unacceptable suffering, and if the particularities of the sacrifice require additional suffering, then solidarity can lose its grip on the moral and social imagination. At that point, more-individualistic, market-oriented approaches become attractive: they make no pretense of solidarity but play directly to self-interest.

However difficult the project, I believe that solidarity must be nurtured as a moral ideal if the provision of equitable health care is to be continued where it already exists, and sought where it does not now exist (as in the United States). If a choice must be made, solidarity is an ideal preferable to, and more plausible than, rights-based claims (though I qualify this point in Chapter 7, on p. 230). But solidarity itself can only be plausible if research medicine reins in its promise of ever-improving life and if patients lower their demands for the relief of suffering. Universal health care and a lively appreciation of individual limits on health care must go together; they require each other. At the same time, solidarity requires a common conviction that disease, illness, and death are our shared problems, even if we suffer them one by one in the privacy of our individual lives. Then, banding together and accepting common limitations, we can develop a medicine that is sustainable.

CHAPTER SIX

Public Health and Personal Responsibility

In the ancient struggle between *hygeia* and *aesculapius*, the scientific victory has mainly gone to *hygeia*. The evidence is now overwhelming that, with a decent environment and sensible health habits, most (but not all) people can live long and healthy lives without much help from medicine.[1] The best prescription for a healthy population is a good public health system, decent jobs and education, and a prudent lifestyle. A comprehensive system of primary care medicine can deal with most of the remaining health problems. I want in this chapter to develop that general case, argue for giving future priority to population health rather than individual health as a way to a sustainable medicine, and show how such an emphasis is perfectly compatible with increased pressure on individuals to live healthier lives.

If the scientific evidence is in favor of the triumph of *hygeia*, why has victory not been declared and a new health regime put in place? Why has there been no replacement for the ancien régime of technological aspiration that has held sway for two centuries, and especially since World War II? The case for public health and personal responsibility as the necessary and almost sufficient foundation for a new, third-era medicine and health care can be made effectively.[2] Making that case logically and scientifically is, unfortunately, the simple part, much easier than capturing public and political support. The obstacles to change are formidable: not only do forces external to health care work against it, but also serious change will have to deal with some other struggles and unresolved tensions.

One matter should be dealt with at once. Precisely because there has been considerable medical progress since the Greeks first developed the distinction between *hygeia* and *aesculapius*, the case for *hygeia* is far stronger now than it was then. *Hygeia* now has the advantage of higher general living standards, supportive medical knowledge, and, for many medical conditions, relatively inexpensive technologies. But as I have tried to show in earlier chapters, the fact that considerable medical progress was made in the past implies neither that it is worth seeking as much progress in the future, nor that it is economically possible to attain as much. Instead, population-oriented health care can help us solidify gains already made, achieve some further affordable gains, and thus lay the foundation for a sustainable medicine. The key to making that possibility plausible is a combination of strong public health and health promotion measures, an expectation and cultural demand that people take better care of themselves, and a judicious, limited use of technology to fill in the gaps.

The Coming Great Struggle:
Public Health and the Market

The great struggle to come, already emerging, is that between public health and personal responsibility, on the one hand, and the market on the other (see Chapter 7). In combination with evidence about the behavioral causes of many illnesses and disabilities, the public health idea has won the scientific struggle—hence my claim for the victory of *hygeia*. But the market idea is coming to win the economic and cultural struggle. Two forces of great weight are thus pitted against each other, the one commanding the inner citadel of health care evidence, the other the political economy of the surrounding countryside.

Now it might perhaps be slightly more accurate to portray a three-way struggle. Is it not the case, possibly, that the real antagonist of a public health approach is reductionistic molecular biology—which seeks the holy grail of *the* causes of disease, and thus the pathway to all cure? The view pits one scientific theory (concerning the socioeconomic determinants of disease) against another (concerning the biological, especially genetic, causes of disease). But it is plausible to see the more important struggle as that between public health and the market for two reasons, even though it pits a scientific against an economic theory. The first is that the evidence for the public health approach is already in hand; it has been gathered and gaining in force for a century. The reductionistic genetics approach is, in contrast, still speculative, and will be beset by many theoretical and practical problems even if the genetic roots of disease can be found. The second reason is more important: it is that the market can, and does already, overshadow both "genetics medicine" and public health. It sets the stage and the social context, and thus has a commanding and still-rising power. The ultimate struggle I have in mind is between the population perspective of public health and the individualist perspective of the market.

Pursuing Public Health

In this chapter I want to lay out both the idea and the ideal of public health, and their role in creating a sustainable medicine. I mean to encompass the following elements, some traditional and some my own: (1) the *scientific view* that the key to population health lies in the background educational, social, economic, and environmental features of society and in the successful deployment of effective health-promotion and disease-prevention programs; (2) the *social ideal*, which understands the struggle against disease, accident, and illness as a matter of solidarity, requiring common effort (for all are mortal) and common sacrifice (for not all needs and desires can necessarily be satisfied) and aiming for a common, collective good health; (3) the *economic conviction* that only a steady-state, economically sustainable medicine oriented to population health ought to be politically acceptable in the future; and (4) the *moral ideal* of a recognition by individuals that their personal behavior will significantly determine their lifetime health prospects and that they have a social obligation to take care of themselves for their own sake as well as that of their neighbor.

With that idea and ideal of public health in hand, I now want to add the final, background colors of a sustainable medicine to the portrait I have sketched in earlier chapters. Our ideas about nature and progress, and our models of medicine, self, and society are, on the whole, important tacit determinants of the way medicine and health care manifest themselves. The more direct vehicles are the ends and means of health care systems, the specific values and techniques used to pursue health. In the case of Western medicine, the background values are these: we give priority to individual patients and to technology and acute-care medicine; we depend heavily upon a rescue commitment, designed to help us once we have become sick; and we share the widespread if usually unspoken belief that medical problems are visited upon people as a matter of fate, not of personal choice or behavior.

The two most important alternatives to that cluster of values are public health, which emphasizes collective rather than individual health, and personal responsibility for health, with its focus on people's choices about how to live. These are the final keys to a sustainable medicine. So what's new? At first sight, they appear to be popular and widely espoused values. Public health has long been touted as a superior way to keep a society well, and the importance of individual health behavior has long been known.

Appearances are highly misleading here. As the scientific case for public health becomes stronger, political and popular support has not kept pace. Public health programs in the United States—and the situation is similar in many other countries—are either not being improved or, in many cases, are being allowed to wither. As the U.S. Department of Health and Human Services noted, between 1981 and 1993 there was a 25 percent decline in funding for public health programs as a proportion of the American health care budget. Some twenty-two state health agencies saw a decline in state funding, and another thirty-three saw cuts to services in 1992. Nothing has improved since then. The state cuts forced local cuts. Disease and injury surveillance, health education, and children's programs have been particularly hard hit.[3]

If public health is a scientific idea whose time has arrived, there is no popular or legislative crowd waving at the station. And while the success of antismoking campaigns in the United States and many countries might suggest that the importance of personal health behavior has finally found its audience, there is continuing resistance to or skepticism about the idea of one's own responsibility in staying healthy in some quarters, and widespread failure to get it taken seriously in most others. Obesity is increasing, exercise declining. The most encouraging sign in the United States is the embrace of health promotion by health maintenance organizations (HMOs).

Yet there are some important tensions, even contradictions, when the public health idea and the personal responsibility ideal are set next to each other, meant to work in tandem. At least part of the public health perspective is that

177

background environmental and sociocultural conditions are the principal determinants of health—that is, health is chiefly influenced not by individual, self-determined behavior but by the setting and context of that behavior. For just that reason, a too-heavy emphasis on individual voluntary behavior is widely opposed in some public health circles as a form of blaming the victim. The real health determinants, it is said, are class, income, educational status, pollution, advertising, profit-seeking, and the like. These are not readily compatible perspectives, and to this tension I will return.

The Case Against a Public Health Strategy

Overt resistance to public health is rare. On the contrary, public health has been subject to the death of a thousand cuts, some of them noticed, others not. The field of public health has sometimes been its own worst enemy, failing to clearly define its function and social place. An important American study of the future of public health had, at the very outset, considerable trouble defining the field, leaving unclear its scope and the way it is to be distinguished from medicine. "The mission of public health [is that of] . . . fulfilling society's interest in assuring conditions in which people can be healthy."[4] That definition does not tell us much and introduces considerable confusion: the "conditions" behind good health cover a considerable range of activities, social as well as medical, and a definition of this kind illuminates little and leaves considerable ambiguity in its wake. Part of the problem with public health in the political arena is surely that it is not well understood, not carefully defined, and thus in the end not well defended.

A more focused definition of public health has been advanced by the U.S. Department of Health and Human Services: "Clinical medicine focuses primarily on caring for and curing existing health problems in individuals; public health focuses on prevention in populations. Clinical medicine devotes its most intensive resources to restoring health or palliating disease in a relatively small number of individuals; public health uses strategies that promote health in large populations, but are not targeted toward any one individual."[5] Three elements appear central to public health: (1) the field focuses on the health of populations as a whole, not the health of individuals; (2) the main goals of the field are, classically, the control of infectious disease and other general hazards to health; health status surveillance and monitoring; and, of late, health promotion and disease prevention; and (3) a central, but not exclusive, role for insuring public health lies with government. My expanded definition of public health, on pp. 175–76, is meant to be compatible with this more common characterization.[6]

How could anyone object to such a respectable set of purposes? Unfortunately, no outright objections are necessary to create obstacles to public health. A widespread set of worries and hesitancies, together with the indifference that sets in when various special interests are not satisfied, does the job nicely. Its focus on the health of populations is enough to get the field off on the wrong foot in an individualistic American culture. Because it is interested in everyone in general but no one in particular, public health necessarily fails to address itself to *my* problems as a particular person. Good public health can and will raise the health status of people as a group, but it will not necessarily help me as an individual. I may be the person who suffers from the chance accident, from lung cancer though I never smoked, from the unchosen genetically wrong parents, from the health problem that stems from unavoidable organ failure, from the idiosyncratic malady—not from the harm done by unhealthy environments, and so on. Generic public health programs do general good, but they may not do individual good except indirectly. That is the inherent political problem with a population-oriented approach to health, which focuses on statistical, not individually identifiable, lives.

Acute-care, high-technology medicine, by contrast, is oriented to dealing with *my* specific problems. It tailors itself to the individual, and in its range of services and skills, can give individuals what they want—if not always what they need—as public health could never do. This situation is exacerbated by our reverence for rescue medicine, the belief that since life is precious any amount of money (and, indeed, almost any injustice to others) is acceptable in preserving it. It is further exacerbated by the traditions of Hippocratic medicine, taken to require the maximum devotion of the physician to individual patient welfare. The public health tradition requiring maximum devotion to population welfare offers a far less attractive approach—however much more it has to recommend it as public policy.

Public health benefits have the further disadvantage that their payoff is usually in the future rather than the present, and the benefits are often unseen. By working to prevent disease, public health chiefly aims to avert what might at some future point happen, not ameliorate what has already occurred. I refer here principally to what is commonly called primary prevention. If public health is successful, something does *not* happen; and that effect is not so easily discerned by its beneficiaries—who may, in any case, not have been present (or even born) when the prevention strategy was put in place. To be sure, public health efforts to curb an epidemic, or to end an outbreak of salmonella, or to find unacceptable bacterial levels in the water supply, will have immediate benefits. But what might be termed the more modern agenda of public health—health promotion and disease prevention—has delayed benefits. Nice—but most of us prefer having rewards and benefits now to having them later. A surgeon who can save my life today is likely to be a more dramatic figure, to whom I will pay larger sums of money, than the public health officer who helps me avoid lung cancer from smoking (which, even without his help, I might not get anyway) thirty years from now.

The Place of Government

Government involvement in public health is suffering a variety of blows around the world. In Asia, particularly in China and Vietnam, rapid privatization is ruining public health programs, which are sinking in the wake of the ships of state that abandon them. In Europe, where the welfare state has less and less power and is accorded less and less respect, public health programs are already threatened, though not so dramatically. In the United States, a more general hostility to government, combined with a drive to hold down the costs of government programs, has weakened federal and state public health programs. Those programs run into general budget-cutting pressures, exacerbated by increased demands for acute-care medicine, which almost always triumphs in the competition for funds. Another problem is that the case for the financial benefits of a public health and health-promotion strategy has not been well made, with good numbers. Confident statements are often made about those benefits, but the available evidence is mixed. This is an issue to which I return below.

There are, in sum, many central features of public health that work against the cultural grain and compete poorly for money. If they do not always lead to direct opposition to public health, they are sufficient to explain the comparative indifference or lack of enthusiasm generated by the field, as well as the foot-dragging that otherwise seems so inexplicable given the favorable outcomes—for instance, reduction in contagious disease, changes in smoking habits, and greater public awareness of good health habits—brought about by public health programs. As if these problems were not enough, the distinguished public health expert Molly Joel Coye has noted a number of additional practical obstacles. Most broadly, public health problems—whether smoking, obesity, lack of exercise, or sexually transmitted disease—combine many elements mediated by behavior and encompass social forces "well outside the 'control' of public health agencies."[7] More specifically, the barriers include ideology or social attitudes (e.g., resistance to government intervention, as demonstrated by the ongoing struggle over motorcycle helmets and opposition by some to public identification of HIV carriers); economic interests (such as the alcohol, firearms, and tobacco industries); and conflicting social goals (freedom of "choice" in smoking versus population health). The separation of medicine and public health into "two distinct cultures," often ignorant of each other, only worsens an already poor situation.[8]

It is important, however, not to paint too dark a picture here. Health screening programs are popular, the Food and Drug Administration (FDA) and the Centers for Disease Control and Prevention (CDC) remain respected and well-supported public agencies, and research on AIDS and TB has sharply increased in recent years, as has support for some education and screening programs. State-level activities in behalf of smoking restrictions, prevention of drunk driving, and gun control have been strong. And mention has already been made of HMO interest in health-promotion efforts. Even so, these are not enough.

The Case Against a Personal Responsibility Strategy

It has been argued that close to half of all premature deaths in the United States are caused by diseases and medical conditions having their origin in unwise, hazardous health behavior.[9] The decrease in death rates from heart disease and stroke, for example, in part can be traced to many helpful behavioral changes in diet and exercise patterns; and great progress has been made in changing smoking behavior, though it took many years to accomplish and has still a long way to go. But after that the success stories begin to thin out. In the United States, obesity has increased; fewer, not more, people exercise regularly; teenage pregnancy remains a stubborn adversary; and distressing evidence has been reported of a resurgence in dangerous sexual behavior by those most at risk for HIV disease. And even in the instance of smoking, moreover, it took evidence (sometimes-disputed evidence) of the effects of passive smoking to bring really strong governmental action, which in turn was met by immediate protest.

Little is really known about how to change unhealthy behavior. Education, in the sense of simply providing information along with mild exhortation, rarely seems sufficient to deal with the most difficult problems. Stronger forms of influence, including economic incentives and disincentives, as well as outright coercion, must run a gauntlet of civil liberties objections from both the left and the right. The cost of effective educational campaigns, moreover, is not inconsiderable.

Yet those worries and objections seem mild in the face of a more enduring set of puzzles and hesitations. It has been exceedingly difficult, first of all, to know how to classify and judge different forms of hazardous behavior. We now penalize smokers, frown on and mildly stigmatize the obese and couch potatoes. But we rarely object to those who practice hang gliding, skydiving, football, mountain climbing, and the like, all of which, though hazardous, are done for recreational and even supposed health purposes and bring pleasure to many people. An effort to devise a consistent set of policies toward dangerous behavior would run afoul of many interest groups, create profound conundrums in evaluating behaviors with mixed outcomes (hazardous forms of recreational exercise, e.g., downhill skiing), and present the threat of a kind of health fascism and preventive zealotry that would probably alienate as many people as it helped.[10]

Much the most far-reaching objection to placing greater responsibility on individuals for their own good health is that, at best, doing so evades the social, environmental, and economic determinants of health, and at worst blames the victim, expecting people to change behavior over which they have little control.[11] An emphasis upon individual responsibility, it is said, allows those responsible for unhealthy social conditions—for instance, lack of jobs, education, and economic mobility; workplace stress—to be released from ultimate culpability for the bad health of those whose lives they dangerously influence. Employers, governments, indifferent fellow citizens can be the real culprits if we seek the true cause of ill health. The question of "cause" itself is disputed and difficult. If cancer can be in part caused by a genetic predisposition, it can be triggered by an unhealthy workplace, and that in turn may reflect conditions of poverty. Where, then, lies the "cause"? What has been called the new health promotion movement wants to shift emphasis away from individual behavior and toward individual social empowerment and community participation in the setting of health goals and identification of health needs. This seems a valuable direction in which to go, although if it is to be effective, it would have to show some change in individual behavior.[12]

Public health research, often excellent at determining the social and economic background patterns of disease, runs into a dilemma when it is used to exhort people to live healthier lives. Public health wants to say that underlying social, economic, and environmental conditions bear heavy responsibility for threats to health and thus are where reform must be focused. But at the same time, public health wants to argue that health promotion campaigns can help persuade people to change unhealthy habits. The problem here is analogous to one sometimes encountered in psychological or psychoanalytical theory: people are understood to be the products of their past, of events well beyond their conscious control; yet they are also expected to learn from insight into that past how to change and be in control of their present behavior.

Many people, using what used to be called willpower, have given up smoking, taken off weight, exercised regularly, and avoided climbing sheer cliffs with no ropes. But many others have not, though they have tried; and even those who succeed are ever subject to relapse. As someone who has been there, along with millions of my fellow creatures, I can testify that it is hard to give up smoking, to drink moderately or not at all, to be constantly vigilant at the dinner table, to exercise on cold, dark nights after a tiring day of work—and to do all this with no guarantee that something else will not strike me down anyway. Wearisome. Boring. Dispiriting. The saints of ancient times lived ascetic lives in order to spend immortality in heaven. We are asked to be secular ascetics, giving up many distinct pleasures so as to qualify for a healthier life and a better death. Is that a fair trade? I hope so. It is not usually an enjoyable one. Asceticism in the name of health does not come easily to most people.

There is also a trap lying in wait for a society that more effectively emphasizes personal responsibility. How can the importance of taking care of one's health be stressed without provoking a counterproductive hypochondria? An extreme sensitivity to health matters, a demand for an absolute reduction of risk, and a drive for a perfect, perfectionistic medicine is already, in the United States, a source of high costs and escalating desires about and demands on health care. Much as any success of the effort to compress morbidity will depend upon swearing off expensive medicine at the end of life, a focus on personal responsibility will somehow have to keep motivation toward healthy behavior from becoming an obsession with health. "Live well" might be the motto, complemented by "Don't be afraid of getting sick." Not an easy combination to promote.

Bringing Public Health and Personal Responsibility Back into Play

I have tried to show that the obstacles and disincentives to a strategy based on either public health or personal responsibility for health are formidable. They are strong enough in recent history to effectively push both approaches to the sidelines, if not necessarily of rhetoric, more importantly of funding and research. Can they be brought back onto the playing field? As matters now stand, they are likely to remain of comparatively small importance unless three conditions are met. The first is that the economic pressures during the waning days of medicine's second era must become intimidating enough that change is mandated whether liked or not. That may already be happening; it helps explain the newfound academic interest in public health strategies (so far not matched by comparable legislative interest, which is where the money is). Yet there is also considerable room left in most health care systems to allow a bit more muddling through, abetted by a variety of cost-controlling measures. Sooner or later, however, pressed by the forces outlined in Chapter 2—aging populations and the intolerable expense of fighting biology at life's margins with technological innovation—the day of reckoning will come.

The second condition is the need to take a long-term view, not expecting quick results. Better that momentum for change, which could well take decades, be initiated immediately than we attempt to put reforms in place at the last minute, which would be difficult and probably ineffective. Now is the time to begin, and it is reasonable to assume that the pressures to do so are already building up at a sufficient rate to make it feasible.

If the background conditions for serious change are important, a positive strategy to force the pace is the third and unavoidable necessary condition. A variety of elements of such a strategy must be put into place: an effective response to the resistance and objections that a combined public health–personal responsibility approach invokes; a way of combining public and private health promotion efforts so that they work effectively together; and a cost-effective use of technology and technological innovation. That innovation can fill in the gaps that will, however good the public health–personal responsibility counterstrategies, inevitably remain even if there is considerable progress toward a new, third era of medicine. All of this must then be orchestrated in a system of medical and health care priorities.

The most important and difficult problem is how to bridge the gap noted above between the seeming abstractness and impersonality of public health medicine—helping everyone in general but not anyone in particular, and insisting that people be responsible for their health—which seems to fly in the face of evidence that many circumstances beyond voluntary control account for poor health. If the public health emphasis seems insufficiently personal, the responsibility emphasis seems too much so.

There is no way to avoid the impersonality of public health. It is not doing its job properly if it pretends to focus on individual health. At the same time, it should be possible to capitalize on some features of the present situation to make the importance of public health more obvious. One of them is the desire, often excessive, to reduce risk. That is what public health can do best and where it has an obvious and distinct advantage over acute-care medicine, which must work after the fact of illness.

Considerably more education about how public health works is important here. The public, interested as individuals in (for instance) not being exposed to unnecessary risk, needs to understand that such a goal can be achieved only by a mixture of population and individually oriented efforts. The wearing of seat belts reduces individual risk even as it requires a personal effort. Safe highways and automobile designs reduce statistical risk to life and limb. Only by working to develop safeguards against dangers to health, and developing information about how to improve or maintain health, can the public health case be made. If that information is combined with other information about the costs of a health care oriented to saving or curing people once sick, a stronger argument can be made for public health.

187

A special hazard at present is that, in the desire to reduce the role and costs of government, programs of health promotion and disease prevention will be relegated to private organizations, particularly managed care companies. These can make a strong contribution to public health, not only by screening and surveillance but also by including disease prevention and health promotion features in their programs. Most are doing just that. But for those efforts to be effective, they must be serious and sustained, and that will depend in great part on whether program managers continue not only to believe that there is a real benefit to subscribers but also that they help to hold down costs. When managed-care programs face sharp competition, health promotion efforts could become the first place where cuts are made. A rapid turnover of plan participants, common in many regions, also discourages health promotion efforts; patients simply don't stay around long enough to promise HMO's a long-term payoff. There is every belief and expectation that managed care can provide both preventive benefits and cost control, but the data collected about the actual results over the next few years are likely to reveal the truth of such claims. At the moment, the issue remains uncertain.[13]

In any event, private managed-care or other insurance programs cannot take the place of strong government programs. They must complement each other. Governments can spot and act on large-scale trends (or sometimes on sickness and infection patterns that are too slight on the local level to be of interest) as private organizations simply cannot. The latter have no special incentive to worry about societal health as a whole, or the health of the uninsured, or regional health patterns that do not particularly affect them. Nor are they likely to have the epidemiological and statistical skills needed to deal well with population health.

The greatest potential contribution of public health is to call attention to the risks of poor health behavior. In its effort to promote health and prevent disease, public health moves from the population to the individual level. Or, better, it focuses attention on the individual determinants of public health, showing how patterns of otherwise private behavior have important aggregate health effects. With respect to this shift from one health arena to another, can the charge be answered that an insistence on individual behavioral change is a way of blaming the victim?

Deserved Blame for the Victim

This question must be answered at two levels. The first level, philosophical, is that of the interaction between individual freedom and those forces operating to diminish freedom or eliminate it altogether. How free are people in the face of strong external pressures? The question whether the human will is free or determined is as ancient as philosophy itself. It is not necessary to take up that vexed matter here, although it might be a good idea to keep in mind an old saying about free will: all theory is against it, all experience favors it.

The second level is that of the actual likelihood that the taking of personal responsibility, even if theoretically possible, can significantly improve population health. On one hand, the evidence is solid that many social and economic circumstances can profoundly affect health. It seems no accident that the poor, those under considerable stress, and those in lower social classes are more prone to disease and disability than those who are better off. It is no less well known that people are influenced in their behavior by advertising, by cultural mores, and by peer pressure; and there are many such pressures working against good health. On the other hand, however, it is evident that people can and do voluntarily change their behavior in the face of those pressures, though often with great difficulty.

Even in those cases where there is real addiction, as with smoking, people can transcend the biological and social pressures to rid themselves of it; and addictions run along a continuum of intensity in any case. That many people fail in such efforts may show one of two things: that individual differences make it harder for some people to manage their behavior than others, or that some people are more responsible about trying to control their unhealthy behavior than others. There is no way of knowing which it is in any particular case, and it is possible that some people are afflicted by both conditions. Unless we invoke some unknown mysterious "factor *x*" to explain why some are unable to control their unhealthy behavior, there is no *evident* reason why they should not be able to do so. The possibility of change should be the working presumption. We may not want to morally blame some whose behavior does not change even though they claim they would like that to happen—but neither can we assume that, because they fail, it is inherently the case that they cannot control their behavior.

Poor background circumstances only increase the probability of bad health behavior. They do not guarantee or compel it. Even though we know that those raised in broken families, beset by poverty, and living in areas rife with crime are more likely to break the law than are those more favorably situated, we do not conclude that they should be released from the demands of the criminal law. Even if life is stacked against them, we still hold them responsible for their actions. We do this in part because it is impossible to show that, because the behavior of *groups* is heavily determined by social circumstance, each individual in the group lacks the freedom to resist those circumstances: not everyone raised in poverty or social chaos lives a life of illness or becomes a criminal.

There is no good reason, therefore, to assume that people are unable to take personal responsibility for their health. It is fallacious to reason that because some people do not overcome their background none can. It seems equally true that if some can do so, others can do so as well. There is an important proviso necessary here. If there is simply no healthful food available, people can hardly be held responsible for their poor eating habits. Nor can it be easy or even possible to exercise— jog, play tennis, swim—in slums where the facilities don't exist to do such things or that are so unsafe that people are afraid to do what might otherwise be possible.

Hence, while I am arguing that people can be expected to act in healthy ways, I recognize that it will be far harder for some than for others, and maybe close to impossible for a few. But for *most* people in reasonably affluent, middle-class circumstances in Western societies, personal responsibility for health is possible, and thus a reasonable social demand. The blame for some smoking can be laid at the feet of to- bacco companies and seductive advertising, just as some obe- sity can be blamed on the pervasiveness of fatty foods and cheap fast-food restaurants. But by no means can most indi- viduals hold themselves blameless because they are subject to those influences. There are thus no good grounds for the ar- gument that to demand that people take care of themselves and live in healthy ways is to blame the victim. Most of the health habits of *most* of us are under our control. We *ought* to be blamed. We are our own worst enemies and the victims of our own choices. At best, we can argue mitigating circum- stances, diminished responsibility, and mild victimization— but only a small minority can claim they lack responsibility altogether.

Yet, as Gerald Dworkin has reminded us, "While it is not *unfair* to treat some people more harshly than others ... whether we *ought* to do so will depend ... [on] how much good we can accomplish and how this can be weighed against other injustices and bad consequences that arise out of the in- stitutions required to implement the policies."[14] It is striking that many European countries have in recent years moved away from even well-established forms of public health coer- cion toward greater voluntariness. A national debate occurred in England when, bucking a European trend in the opposite direction, mandatory immunization of children for a variety of infectious diseases was instituted in the last few years.[15]

Blameworthy Victims, Recalcitrant Behavior

Even if there are poor empirical and philosophical grounds for arguing that people cannot be responsible for their health, is it not simply naive to think it possible to change harmful behavior in any widespread way? "Is it too much," John Powles asked in 1973, "to expect a . . . future interaction between specific advice on changing damaging health habits and a wider culture which is increasingly sensitive to the need . . . to treat the natural world with respect?"[16] Some people have indeed made just that connection in their daily lives—but mainly affluent, comfortable people. Can it spread to others less well situated? Nice philosophical arguments rarely change the way people live and act. Smoking is one place where real change has been accomplished, and it has taken the assistance of the law to bring that about.

Yet for all its singularity, the decline in smoking does show the sequence of events necessary to bring about a meaningful change. There must first be good evidence of a serious risk to health, and at least some evidence to suggest that there can be harm to others as well; a strong, government-led program to call attention to the dangers and to institute educational efforts; a portion of the citizenry that takes up the cause with great zeal; a turning to the law to accomplish what persuasion cannot achieve on its own; and, finally, a widespread repugnance at the practice, supported by the combined force of law, public opinion, civic shaming, stigmatization, and a critical mass of people who do not indulge in the behavior and will not tolerate it in others. And we should not overlook the fact that although those conditions have been met, many people continue to smoke, and young people take it up much as they did in the past (even if they apparently do not persist as long as earlier generations did). Yet even incomplete and imperfect behavioral change can represent a great triumph, decisively altering health outcomes.

Can something comparable be achieved with respect to other conditions? Not easily. Apart from smoking, few other health hazards are as accessible to pressure and the force of law. Bad diet and lack of exercise are not subject to legal surveillance the way smoking is. We cannot ban eating in fast-food restaurants, or punish a refusal to walk when a car is available, or ostracize those who lie too long in front of television sets (especially when educational programs are on). The kind of discrimination we now widely and gleefully practice against smokers, has, when tried with the obese, led to charges of unfair discrimination and the reply that, perhaps, obesity is somehow genetically caused and therefore that any public discrimination or private scorn is unfair, even grossly so. I find that argument unpersuasive—genetic predispositions alone cannot determine behavior—but the fact that it is used in an organized way suggests the difficulty of bringing about behavioral change.

Carrots and Sticks

Is health promotion, then, simply to be left to the relatively ineffective methods of education, occasional legislation, and circumspect cajolery? Not necessarily. More effective means can be devised, but only after three basic questions have been answered:

First, is the evidence in favor of the efficacy of taking personal responsibility for health strong enough to place it beyond reasonable doubt? If people could change their unhealthy habits, would that make a great difference in their personal health outcomes? I believe the answer is yes, and decisively so.[17]

Second, would the combined force of many individuals

193

changing their health habits have an important collective benefit, reducing the overall burden of individual and societal illness and making a measurable difference in national health care costs? I believe the answer to that question is a hesitant yes, keeping in mind a number of controversies and disagreements on the economic benefits.[18] On balance, the conflicting evidence and arguments seem to suggest that health promotion and public health efforts by no means automatically save money. They can sometimes increase costs and can show a poor cost-benefit ratio. However, *in general* they seem a cost-effective way to spend health care money, which also produces additional social benefits.

Third, would the individual and social benefits of serious efforts to change behavior warrant strong, even severe, intrusions upon personal liberty? My answer to that question is guarded, though I believe the time has come for an extended and serious public and professional debate on the topic.[19] There are many moral and practical objections to coercing health-related behavior—potential invasions of privacy, infringements of liberty, unfair judgments of others, and so on. Yet if we are not, *as a society*, able to take strong steps to change unhealthy behavior, the provision of adequate health care will become increasingly difficult, bringing about far harsher, albeit indirect, intrusions upon liberty. There will, in particular, be a decline in the present liberty to enjoy poor health habits, confident that medicine will come to the rescue. That will be less possible in the future, especially for the elderly.

While the first two questions are factual, bearing on what we know of the benefits of greater personal responsibility, the third question is, of course, moral and political. To make the case for the legitimacy of strong, even coercive, interventions into the personal sphere in the name of health, some particular conditions need to be met: a serious and demonstrable harm to the community must be at stake; the harm done to individual welfare by behavioral intervention must be relatively

194

slight and transitory, and the interventions not in themselves harmful; and the interventions must be practically and legally feasible. Seat belt laws and laws mandating motorcycle helmets and (for children) bicycle helmets meet those criteria; the need now is to find other, equally valid interventions. If it is becoming financially more difficult to practice expensive rescue medicine, then there is every incentive to look for ways to change unhealthy behavior.

In addition to the need to meet the criteria mentioned above, such interventions will have to meet some additional political conditions. One of them is that a decision to coerce private behavior has been reached by democratic means, that is, by achieving the collective support of the community whose behavior is to be coerced. The coercion must, that is, be self-imposed by the community, much as the current restrictions on the liberty to smoke have been imposed by duly elected and authorized officials. Of course, not everyone will welcome this coercion, but that is true of many other democratically achieved limitations on liberty. The other condition is that the restrictions and coercions do not violate any fundamental human rights, do not impose insupportable burdens, and do not do collateral harm to those whose liberty is denied. As we know, of course, motorcyclists have effectively lobbied in many states to have helmet laws repealed; the political process does not always favor healthy behavior. Yet there is no choice but to rely upon it.

Despite the "pro-choice" arguments of, say, the National Smokers Alliance, I know of no claimed right of individuals to threaten the welfare of society by unhealthy behavior.[20] Laws against spitting, urinating, and defecating in public places have public health as their principal goal, and are well accepted in all civilized societies. It is now time to move on to still more areas of private activity. Unhealthy private behavior, even if hidden from the public eye, can have equally harmful public consequences: excessive obesity and lack of exercise increase the health care costs of all, while teenage pregnancy generates myriad undesirable social and familial harms. For that matter, a person who lives an egregiously unhealthy private life is more likely to do harm to us (and his family) through his health care burdens and costs than someone who urinates on the sidewalk. It is cheaper to hose down a sidewalk than to subsidize ICU care.

In modern, interdependent societies, and in modern health care systems, where risks and costs are shared, the private realm quickly affects the public realm. Everything we do to ourselves behind closed doors, from sex to diet to exercise, will have a public impact. While it is difficult, in free societies, to find a legal or moral basis to coerce competent adults for their own good, it may be possible to make such a case on social grounds—that is, the effect of our unhealthy behavior on others, directly (as with passive smoke) or indirectly (shared community costs of health care).[21]

There is a unique feature of coercive efforts to change unhealthy behavior: save for damage done to the liberty of those we socially coerce, no direct physical harm is done to them. If the evidence is strong that the health of individuals is likely to be improved in the absence of bad health behaviors, then the health benefits of coercion will be direct and unassailable. Our social coercion will be good for them and good for the rest of us. But what about the psychological harm done to those whose apparent needs and desires are thwarted? The most plausible response to that question is this: does anyone have evidence that obese people denied unhealthy diets suffer irreparable psychological damage, or that daily moderate exercise leads to emotional breakdown, or that an inability to smoke indoors destroys many lives?

These rhetorical questions, unfortunately, will not readily overcome a resistance to coercion. Do we not have a right, many would ask, to use our bodies as we see fit, healthfully or unhealthfully as the case may be? Yes, but only up to a point— when there is proof that harm is done to others by what we do to ourselves. Such harm does not, however, often meet the naked eye. Bad individual health behavior, in an interdependent health care system (and there is no other kind) does harm to others, even if the health risk-takers pay their own health care costs. Money is diverted from other uses, personnel are diverted from other patients, and lives are wasted that could serve all of us. Moreover, a sustainable medicine, based on social solidarity as a core value, requires that we take account of the impact of individual behavior, the burdens we impose on each other, directly or indirectly, by our health behavior, and the need to find nontechnological ways of improving health.

A theoretical case might, therefore, be made for forceful interventions into unhealthy behavior as a way to a sustainable medicine. A showing of some direct harm, or burden, to others could be sufficient. Yet even if we could agree in principle, it is by no means easy to see how to develop the public policy and accompanying regulations that would effectively, justly, and prudently coerce people into better health. A number of stiff public policy tests would have to be passed to make the coercion acceptable (my standard of "psychologically sustainable"). They include developing policies that can ensure compliance and efficacy, that can show the communal benefits outweighing the individual burdens, that can minimize and render transitory the harm done to the individuals coerced, and that will in the end and in fact significantly improve population health. This is an exceedingly heavy set of burdens to discharge and probably explains why the police powers of public health systems have been invoked only in times of contagious plagues and epidemics, where the harm to a population is grievous, immediate, and visible to all.

While the economic and social burden of much harmful contemporary health behavior may be as great, in statistical terms, as many ancient plagues (surely the case with tobacco-induced illness), the results are not so evident or immediate and thus far harder to cope with. This makes it all the easier to invoke civil liberties objections to coercion and to stress the uncertainty of success even if coercion is used (think of trying to control teenage pregnancy this way), and all the more difficult to demonstrate immediately foreseeable economic benefits. Nonetheless, however difficult and distasteful, coercion is a necessary course to pursue at times, forcefully but carefully.

What are some of the possible techniques of incentives and coercive interventions that might be employed? An approach already used on occasion by some employers and insurers is to charge higher premiums for those who, say, smoke or are significantly overweight. A denial of benefits for those who injure themselves as a result of such reckless behavior as drunken driving has been successfully employed in at least one case. Predictions have been made that managed-care programs may come to require that their members pay part of their costs if they neglect their health. Managed-care programs could, as stated policy, require participation in health promotion programs and health risk monitoring. Such practices are now ordinarily voluntary; there is no reason, save for employee protest, why they could not be made mandatory. Of course such mandatory practices could face legal challenges. That possibility, plus the damage to employee morale or the public image of employers, is probably sufficient at the moment to make most employers hesitate to go that far. In the end, as the philosopher Haavi Morreim has noted, "The value of greater economic accountability for patients is found not in its power to change their lifestyles, but in its capacity to foster more responsible use of health care resources generally, [and] to return to patients a greater measure of control over their health care."[22]

As the Morreim approach suggests, only economic and related incentives are likely to do any good and to be socially and legally acceptable. While legal sanctions have been effective in the case of smoking, they will, in general, be unavailable with other forms of poor health behavior: diet, exercise, sexual behavior. Even if such sanctions were socially and legally tolerable, it is difficult to see how they could be effectively enforced. A policeman in every obese person's kitchen?

Hardly. Even in the more serious case of AIDS, there is little that the law can do to stop risky behavior. Bathhouses can be closed, but they are not where the largest problem arises—in ordinary sexual contacts.

As the health lawyer George Annas has suggested, "Protecting liberty and protecting public health simultaneously can almost always be accomplished by concentrating on making things (rather than people) safer."[23] While I am not as optimistic as Annas that there need be no conflict between public health and personal liberty, there seems little doubt that public health can politically and legally be promoted by stressing liberty, and that extensive coercive policies or regulations will probably not pass public opinion scrutiny in the immediate future. Even so, a sustainable medicine will require an effective continuum of programs of public health, health promotion, and disease prevention, a continuum ranging from education at one end of the spectrum, economic and other incentives in the middle, and some frankly coercive policies at the other end. Education alone, or education and exhortation, cannot do the necessary work. Coercive programs will be necessary, and research and public debate with that end in mind now seems imperative.

One form of coercion in the name of health should never be tolerated, however: the ex post facto punishment or penalization of those whose bad health behavior has—allegedly or actually—led to their illness or disability. The most ancient and important traditions of medicine hold that the sick are to be treated regardless of the cause of the sickness or the culpability of the afflicted person. The dangers of tinkering with, or putting aside, those traditions are enormous. Our physician would become our moral judge as well as our healer, and the judge might decide not to heal, just as those who pay for health care may correspondingly decide not to care. The possibilities of error and injustice would be great and unavoidable. The only acceptable form of coercion must come when people are still well, when they have a chance to do something about their health behavior and can be penalized before, not after, the fact of harm. A punitive medicine would be fearful.

I would suggest one final incentive, in the form of a sobering thought to be put before today's young and middle-aged people: you are almost certainly not going to receive benefits in your old age, in the years 2015 to 2040, comparable to those now received by the present elderly, your parents and grandparents. Not only are businesses reducing, even eliminating, once-generous retirement programs, the coming projected deficits in the Medicare program for the aged, now reasonably bountiful in its medical benefits, guarantee a sharp reduction of those benefits in the future. Just as the present younger generation has now come to understand that their government Social Security benefits will not be generous or solid, and that a campaign of personal savings to supplement Social Security is not only prudent but imperative, so also they should assume a decrease in medical benefits, and begin developing those health habits conducive to good health in old age. What I am suggesting here requires no coercive incentives at all, just a persistent, and widely publicized, appeal to self-interest and common sense. The present American health care system, quite apart from my more utopian sustainable medicine, will not be able to provide lavish benefits to the future elderly. So: Take care of yourself. Get ready for limits. Prepare for rationing. That should be the message.

Crafting Policy for a Sustainable Medicine

In all of this, as ways are sought to change poor health behavior, moderation and common sense would be imperative. Any coercion, economic or otherwise, would have to be careful and measured, not oppressive. It would contradict my plea for a more moderate view of the importance of health in society—health is a good, but not the supreme human good—to support a health fundamentalism, a Calvinism of the body, justifying the most draconian measures to force people to live more salubrious lives. "Will we," Dr. Faith Fitzgerald has asked, "speak of people as innocent victims only when we can, after thorough exploration, find nothing in their lifestyles to account for their disabilities? And if health involves not only physical disarray but also emotional and social disarray, how far will we go in establishing laws to regulate 'healthy behavior,' arguing that it is for the individual's own good as well as for the public good?"[24]

A Big Brother society in the name of health is no more palatable than one established in the name of political conformity or economic advancement; and it obviously works against the psychological sustainability needed to gain public acceptance. Moreover, as noted earlier, it may well be that because of economic and social circumstances or genetic predispositions, excessive coercion could be patently unfair to some people. Even with those to whom such an effort would not be unfair, the obstacles to gaining sufficient acceptance, even with supportive laws, would be significant. There can be no doubt, therefore, that coercive strategies would generate both moral and practical dilemmas, which should not be minimized (and surely offer one reason why they have never widely been used).

There is only one way out of this dilemma. We will need a clever combination of efforts to change the economic and social circumstances conducive to poor health, and, at the same time, broad educational efforts and a variety of moderate and measured incentives, a few coercive, designed to change individual behavior.[25] To the charge that incentives and coercion would be tantamount to blaming the victim, the only acceptable response would be to show that we not only assume the possibility of free choice but are also making efforts to deal with those conditions that rob people of meaningful choice. "Health promotion efforts," the public health expert Meredith Minkler has noted, "which fail to address the social context within which people live not only minimize the possibility of success, but also risk violating the ethical admonition to 'do no harm.'"[26] To the charge that it is impossible, as a practical matter, to wholly change background circumstances, the responses should be that individuals are capable, despite those circumstances, of changing behavior if appropriate incentives are in place to push them in that direction. The worry that Theodore Marmor and his colleagues have voiced about the likely failure of "individual exhortation and collective regulation of behavior" to challenge those "traditional structures of power" responsible for work, income distribution, and control over the environment must be heeded.[27] If the end result of such a challenge is to reach the individual, it would be a mistake simply to begin with the individual, acting as if his or her behavior were not influenced by a wide range of background conditions.

Moreover, it would, in any case, hardly be necessary for everyone to behave sensibly in order to improve the health status of a society more generally. The aim would be overall improvement, not a perfect victory. The Intersalt study of health patterns has shown that, when the overall health behavior of a society is good, deviations from the norm are less likely. By contrast, when everyone is heavier, obesity is more common, and when everyone drinks a good deal, alcoholism will be more pervasive. Not only, then, is there a subtle correlation, perhaps causal, between the way most of us act and the way some, deviantly, act, there is an even more interesting implication: "We will not succeed in solving any large array of societal and health-related problems . . . as long as we concentrate on those individuals who deviate from the majority. . . . We will have to change the behavior of the majority. . . . The influence we have on one another is not limited to a small circle of acquaintances."[28] Medicine has not been, and will not be, able to overcome external nature; it will not wholly be able to overcome the recalcitrance of human nature, either. Yet there is so much room for improvement in general health behavior, and so many social and individual reasons to pursue it, that the potential contribution to a sustainable medicine is considerable.

A Sustainable Complementary Technology

A strategy that would combine enhanced public health programs with pressure on people to better manage their health behavior would require one other obvious ingredient. It would have to have available the range and kind of technology that would enhance the gains achieved and, at the same time, fill in the gaps that neither public health measures nor personal responsibility can do much about. We will all be subject to accidents, no matter how careful we are; we will all be subject to the genetic lottery; and our finite, imperfect bodies will insist on getting sick from time to time no matter what we do. Most important, we will all get old and the diseases and debilities of age will eventually get us all. *Aesculapius* will always rightly claim his day. We will inevitably turn to technology to deal with those problems, and nothing I have written so far should be construed as a brief for getting rid of technology. That is not the issue. The problem is how to find and support a *level* and *kind* of technology that will neither seek a total victory over nature, nor seek perfection or the elimination of all risk, nor do more than round off the natural biological life cycle of human beings, nor financially beggar us.

I will outline here some suggested principles for a sustainable technology, to complement the public health and personal-responsibility strategies.[29] They are what I will call the principles of communal sufficiency, minimal individual adequacy, and technological economy.

1. Communal Sufficiency. A sustainable medicine and its accompanying technology will provide a community with a level of health sufficient for that community to function well and to provide its members with a fair chance at an adequate life in the community. The task of providing this sufficiency will fall to government or to those mechanisms determined culturally most suitable; these might be some combination of governmental and employer programs. The point of an emphasis on sufficiency is that there can be no pretense of a guarantee that everyone, regardless of condition, will get everything they might individually need. It will be the task of government to ensure that the community has what, in general, it needs to keep the majority of its citizens healthy, not what would be required to keep each and every one healthy. The aim is to overcome the present assumption that health care should be tailored to individual needs, an approach that must rely on technology to do what public health and personal responsibility cannot do.

Communal sufficiency will include an effort to help the majority of citizens avoid premature death, and to protect them from epidemics, contaminated food and water, correctable environmental hazards, and the like. Technologies for this purpose should have the highest priority. The primary function of technology in helping to enhance communal sufficiency will be to allow useful monitoring, screening, and health promotion and disease prevention programs—that is, the technology will be oriented toward public and not individual health. Educational programs using the best available communication technologies and designed to help individuals maintain good health will be imperative here.

2. *Minimal Individual Adequacy.* If communal sufficiency is to be given priority, room must still be made for individual need, a secondary but still important priority. Every person has a reasonable claim on society—in the name of the common good and solidarity, not individual rights—to receive a minimally adequate level of individual medical care. The level of care should build on public health efforts and on programs aimed at educating people how to stay in good health (and sometimes

coercing them to do so). The overriding aim will not be to meet each and every health and medical need, but only those that are most common.[30] Interventions in childhood may be particularly effective and comparatively inexpensive, laying a solid foundation for later life.[31] I develop these points further in Chapter 8.

A sustainable medicine requires equal access to basic services, not an equal health outcome. It is precisely the pursuit of the latter through medical perfectionism or the reduction of all risks that contributes heavily to an unsustainable medicine. Sustainable medicine's main goals will be to help most people avoid a premature death and, when they are old, to provide primary and palliative care, not the means to avoid all possibilities of death. Since a principal aim of sustainability will be an affordable medicine, once the public health and primary care needs have been met the next-highest priority should go to technologies that reduce morbidity and disability, helping people to remain independent and self-sustaining. When that is no longer possible, long-term care, home care, and palliative medicine become important. The lowest priority should be given to those conditions that affect comparatively few people and require significant expenditures or technology.

Minimal individual adequacy will be achieved when most people have a statistically high probability of receiving over their lifetime the kind and amount of health care they need to survive and to function at the levels common in their society. These standards mean, I stress, that *some* people — those who fall outside the general statistical probabilities, or who have unusual conditions, or whose care is excessively expensive — will not fare as well as their neighbors. These are the implications of a population-based health care strategy: it runs risks to individuals, works against expensive marginal technologies, and is willing to accept unequal health outcomes for some (though through chance, not through deliberate discrimination).

3. *Technological Economy.* The most important research top-
ics in the years ahead will be how to strengthen public health
programs, how to improve health and prevent disease, and
how to motivate people to engage in healthy behavior. Technologies that can enhance those possibilities should have a
high priority. Low-cost technologies to help the elderly, the
fastest-growing part of the population, should have a special
priority.[32] At the same time, technologies that benefit comparatively few people at a high cost should have lower priority, as should those that provide only marginal gain at a high
cost. General research efforts to reduce the causes of death in
old age should have the lowest priority, as should efforts to
provide to elderly populations life-extending technologies.
Here as elsewhere, medical perfectionism and efforts to eliminate all risk pose the greatest hazards to a sustainable medicine and health care system.

Medical technology should become an adjunct to the
public health system, reserved for those medical conditions
in which only a technological intervention can preserve
health. Given a recent history of technologies that in the
main have increased costs rather than decreased them, and
have done so without a great improvement in overall health
status, the emphasis should fall on the development of inexpensive technologies designed to serve large numbers of people. We should discourage technologies that will increase
costs with comparatively little population benefit. The question in the future is not whether a technology will serve *some*
people—not a hard standard to meet—but whether it will
help *most* people by addressing conditions of which most
people will be at risk, and in a way that can show community,
not just individual, benefit.

The rationing of health care will be a part of any and all
health care systems. The place to begin that rationing is with
expensive, high-technology rescue medicine, a principal ingredient in the costs of contemporary health care.[33] Emphasis

should instead be placed on developing technologies that can work to keep people well in the first place. When that fails, the available technologies should be sharply limited to those with the best population benefits, and those that provide comfort and palliation.

CHAPTER SEVEN

Can This Marriage Succeed? Medicine and the Market

It is a rare event when an idea pronounced dead, its last rites already said, manages to revive itself, ringing the bell in its coffin so insistently that the lid is raised for another look. This has been the good fortune of the idea of "the market," seemingly killed off in Europe and in some American circles by the early twentieth century, but now alive once again, and perhaps all the stronger for having come back from the grave, as if its temporary out-of-body existence allowed a fresh heavenly vision and it was only awaiting its chance to become incarnate in actual societies. That chance came in Europe with the collapse of the Communist countries of Eastern Europe, with the thinning of the blood of the welfare state and democratic socialism in Western Europe, and with the revival of conservative thought and politics in the United States. The American development brought together a hostility to government and a celebration of the power of choice, that notion so congenial to both liberals and conservatives as the twentieth century winds down.

Medicine and health care have, like most other institutions, been caught up in this triumphant market revival. They seem ripe candidates indeed. With the possible exception of welfare and Social Security provisions, no other sector of society has proved to be such a financial burden, so relentlessly subject in recent years to costs that have outrun inflation and to public demand for more and better health care that only rises as that care improves. Neither the European welfare state nor the tattered American safety-net state has been able effectively to cope with so insistent a drive for improved health care. What is to be done?

The market, back among the living, offers itself as the answer to that question. Its attractive promissory note is that it will deal efficiently and toughly with the cost-inflationary pressures of medicine and, by putting more choice into the hands of patients, simultaneously satisfy the demands of freedom and the need for economic discipline. Government and the market can, moreover, effectively help each other.[1] The market offers, in short, not just an answer to some problems of medicine and health care, but a comprehensive answer to most of them. That is an ambitious claim, with a great deal of its force lying in the positive hope of something better and in the negative prod of moving away from a variety of welfare-state models that seemingly fail the test of economics.

The contention of the previous chapter was that only (a) a population-oriented health policy, combined with (b) a strong emphasis on personal responsibility and working hard for (c) reduced dependency upon technological medicine, would be sufficient to bring about a sustainable medicine. At various points in the book I have pointed a finger at the market and the commercialization of health care as a cause—but by no means the only cause—of an unsustainable medicine. Nonetheless, not the least of the reasons for the attractions of the market is that, by virtue of its drive for profitable innovation and the satisfaction of needs and desires, it provides a number of benefits, medical and economic, social and individual. A more recent and potent factor, an ironic outcome of that situation, is an increased reliance on the market to bail governments out of unwanted and unaffordable support of health care. The market, a source of medicine's problems from one direction (helping to create an unaffordable medicine) is then looked to, from another direction, as the answer to those problems (by privatization or market incentives, for instance). Nonetheless, if the outcome of a move to the market is an unsustainable medicine, then the net result is nothing less than a communal disaster, even if many individuals and some sectors of the community are better off.

Now, while I believe that judgment to be true as a general thesis, realism demands two important concessions and, concomitantly, the development of a modus vivendi between medicine and the market. The first concession is that the idea of "the market" is complex and that if, in general, medicine in toto and the market in toto cannot make a happy marriage, some elements of market thinking and strategy can be useful for achieving a sustainable medicine. The other concession is that, given the present difficulties that governments have in paying for health care, the market will inevitably be turned to as a way out. It thus seems to me fruitless simply to point out the incompatibility of medical and market ideals, and then to condemn the market out of hand. That will do no good. A more serious need is to see if they can work together more productively. The aim of this chapter will be, first, to analyze in a general way the problems posed when efforts are made to marry medicine and the market; and second, to offer some ways out of those problems, solutions that can contribute to a sustainable medicine.

Medicine and the Market

In Book I of the *Republic*, Plato wrote: "The physician, as such, studies only the patient's interest, not his own. . . . The business of the physician, in the strict sense, is not to make money for himself, but to exercise his power over the patient's body. . . . All that he says and does will be said and done with a view to what is good and proper for the subject for whom he practices his art."[2] This perception is in obvious contrast to that classical text of the market, Adam Smith's 1776 contention in *Wealth of Nations* that "It is not from the benevolence of the butcher, the brewer, or the baker, that we expect our dinner, but from their regard to their own interest."[3] Taken alone, of course, these two texts are not quite parallel. Historically, the doctor has often served his self-interest, financial and otherwise; and the butcher and the baker have served the needs of our bodies as well as of their purses. But the main point is that medicine has been thought of, by its nature, to be directed away from self-interest.

Given their histories and starting points, can there be a successful marriage between medicine and the market? But that is only part of the full struggle. Medicine is already caught up in the war between the individualism of the market—which sets choice, efficiency, and competition as its highest virtues and resolutely puts aside formal visions of a collective moral good—and the communitarianism of government-run welfare states—which, one way or another, have some model in mind of the common good.

There is also a struggle between the market and the public health ideal. The market model offers a direct challenge to the public health ideal, overcoming the disadvantage I earlier noted of the population approach—that of helping everyone in general but no one in particular. The market is oriented to individual wants, as defined by patients themselves (and their

211

doctors), not to population health. The market is quite happy to see constant technological innovation, both because people patently want it for their individual benefit and because, when all is said and done, there is no reason why a desire for profits and a good living should not be generated by medicine. The market has no reason to encourage either a public health or a personal-responsibility approach, much less both together. And that is the rub. The principal liability of a market bias in health care, as I will develop, is its severe threat to economic sustainability, at least at an affordable psychological price.

In his provocative book *The Two Cultures and the Scientific Revolution*, the late C. P. Snow deplored the relationship between science and the humanities, excoriating in particular the ignorance of science displayed by most humanists.[4] If there have always been gaps between the sciences and the humanities, they seem slight in comparison with that between medicine and economics. Here is a tale of two cultures now being forced together, but whose starting points and spirit could hardly seem more dissimilar.[5] Medicine has, to be sure, never scorned money or a certain degree of commerce. Doctors have lived well when they could; London's Harley Street physician, catering to the rich and fashionable, and his Park Avenue colleague in New York, find their counterpart in almost every society. The great jump in the income of physicians that marked the 1960s and 1970s in the United States, and that saw the emergence of a popular journal, *Medical Economics*, devoted to helping doctors increase their income, met no resistance from physicians and only a little from the general public.

Yet there is an enormous difference between a discipline and profession whose practitioners do not resist the personal good life when it comes their way, and one which has that life as its purpose. Medicine has always professed to be, and has mainly been, an institution whose dominating focus has been health and the healing of sick persons. It is in that sense philanthropic at its core, seeking not the good of its practi-

212

tioners but the good of those it serves. It rests on a moral foundation of compassion and the relief of suffering as a high calling. It has always condemned those doctors who would put their own good, financial or otherwise, ahead of their patients'. In the pursuit of health and the postponement of death, the goals of medicine have looked outward to the good of others, not inward.

I will not say more here about the culture of medicine. More pertinent at this stage of my argument is the culture of the market and the way that culture affects medicine. While the history of medicine and the market—particularly in their post–World War II phase—has yet to be written, I suggest that the following encouraging ingredients will be seen as crucial, though the proportions might vary from country to country:

- the emergence of effective medicine, sharply increasing public demand

- the growth of the pharmaceutical and medical-equipment industry, which came to see an enormous profit potential in postwar medicine

- the simultaneous increase in the relative cost of good medicine, as cures, therapies, and diagnostic procedures increased at a rapid rate

- the growing inability of individuals to pay for good medical care out of their own pockets, bringing government in as a primary organizer and provider of health care in most countries and turning health care into an important public activity everywhere

- the greater pressures on physicians and other health care workers to receive a complex, lengthy, and expensive training, able to keep them informed and up-to-date in an ever-changing technological landscape

- an intensification of the romance of progress and constant innovation, fed by professional and public demand and commercial profit

- the subsidization by government of medical schools and teaching hospitals

- the growing cost of effective medicine to deal with the problems of chronic disease and aging societies, the result of the earlier success of medicine.

If the market was gradually brought into medicine because of this combination of forces, it did not at first have the status of an ideology, or the set of values that it has taken on in recent years. That result was produced by a combination of the gross failure of the Communist states, including most conspicuously their health care systems, and the increasing strain on governments everywhere (and on employers in many countries) in trying to keep pace with the costs of medicine. The market, a minor though growing force up through the 1960s, became "The Market" and a major force in the 1970s and 1980s, but especially in the 1990s.

The Culture of the Market

To speak at all of the culture of the market may seem strange. Unlike medicine, the market is not an institution. Its followers and practitioners have no mandatory educational requirements, its professionals take no equivalent of the Hippocratic Oath (it is not clear just who those professionals are, anyway), and it does not take comfortably to the language of a specific human good (other than, perhaps, that of general prosperity). What is the market, then? A standard dictionary definition is that it is "an exchange mechanism that brings together sellers and buyers of a product, factor of production, or financial security."[6] That does not tell us much. The market is best thought of, I believe, in its widest sense as an ensemble of means and techniques of exchange for the pursuit of individual or corporate economic self-interest, with an attendant assumption that that pursuit will be of indirect collective benefit, whether to small or large groups.

At present, the market's motive force in medicine and health care is varied: to help government reduce its economic burden by shifting more financing and provision into private hands; to control costs, whether public or private; to increase efficiency; to maximize individual choice; and to encourage managerial, communicative, and technological innovation. If the flavor and strategies of market use are different in Europe—emphasizing "the market as policy adjustment"—that is, as a tool to be used mainly by government officials—it has much the same perceived utility as in the United States: principally, to control costs, increase efficiency, and relieve government burdens.[7]

To achieve these ends, the market brings to bear a characteristic set of methods. As Maurizio Ferrara has nicely laid out, these methods include a managerial (innovative, entrepreneurial) rather than bureaucratic (rigid, hierarchical) style in the organization of services; the promotion of cost-conscious behavior by the "consumers" of health care (a.k.a. patients) through the introduction of copayment arrangements and new systems of remuneration (e.g., negotiation with doctors); the stimulation of competition and other characteristic market-type interactions between purchasers and providers; the outright and deliberate expansion of the private market for health care; and, of critical importance, the establishment of tougher criteria for access to government universal-care programs, thus watering down the ideal of democratic universalism in the provision of health care.[8]

Where medicine as a historical institution has a specific human value—health—as its focus, the market as an assemblage of techniques is meant to be applicable to a wide range of human activities. A common claim of market proponents is that market techniques can be used in activities not specifically economic in nature, but where economic considerations—and especially scarcity of resources—are important. Such endeavors include education, transportation, and housing, for instance—any activity, that is, in which competitive economic and other incentives, together with the harnessable power of self-interest, come into play. At the same time, as Daniel Sarewitz has observed, "the economic frame of reference interprets progress as the enhanced ability of individuals to pursue options, opportunities, and desires."[9]

In the (rather remarkable) absence of any clear consensus on the nature and limits of the market, I find it helpful to think of the idea of the market as combining three parts: a theory of human nature; a view of the dynamics of human behavior; and a political philosophy.

The Market and Human Nature

The view of human nature underlying much market theory is that people are fundamentally self-interested; this is held to be simply a fact of that nature and thus a reasonable starting point for organizing economic relationships. A decently working society will be one that allows people to maximize rationally their self-interest. But this idea can be taken in different directions, and there are competing views of the market, human nature, and morality.

One common view of the eighteenth-century origin of the market idea, in Adam Smith, was that a market economy would and should be created on top of a society already bound together by a strong underlying societal morality. The economist Amartya Sen has pointed to the failure of many readers of Adam Smith to notice "his observations on misery, the need for sympathy, and the role of ethical considerations in human behavior [and] particularly the use of behaviour norms."[10] The

216

sociologist Alan Wolfe has underscored the same point: "Only by preserving a realm of morality against all instrumentalism, including the instrumentalism of economic calculation itself, could a society be free to allow economic calculation to take place. . . . From precapitalist traditions there developed an emphasis on self-restraint, charity, and the organic unity of society that held to a minimum the damage caused by the pursuit of self-interest. From the postcapitalist ideology of the welfare state there developed a concern for solidarity, protection of the weak, and the organic unity of society that filled in the moral gap at just about the time that religions, community, and family bonds weakened."[11]

As Adam Smith himself once wrote, "No society can be flourishing or happy, of which the far greater part of its members are poor and miserable. It is but equity, besides, that they who feed, cloath [sic] and lodge the whole body of the people should have such a share of the produce of their own labor as to be themselves tolerably well fed, cloathed and lodged."[12] Is it too great a historical leap to imagine that Smith would have extended this conviction to late-twentieth-century health care, and particularly to the 41 million uninsured Americans, most of whom are employed?

But there is another, competing, view of the market. For the so-called Chicago school, led by Milton Friedman, George Stigler, and Gary Becker, there is no behavior that cannot be reduced to economic behavior. As Becker, a Nobel laureate, has put it, "The economic approach is uniquely powerful because it can integrate a wide range of human behavior."[13] "Man," George Stigler has written, in defending the view that self-interest explains all human behavior, "is eternally a utility maximizer . . . in his church, in his scientific work, in short, everywhere."[14] This belief sets the stage for an application of the market to all human activities, including morality itself, thereby erasing that understanding of the market which builds economic activity on the moral limits set by underlying cultures. Viable cultures promote solidarity and self-restraint, and thus offer a standing counterbalance to excessive and destructive economic self-interest. But for the Chicago school, that restraint is in principle removed.

I will not try to decide which interpretation of the market, human nature, and culture is most true to the historical market idea; both have their adherents. It is only important to note that a self-interest constrained by counterbalancing moral values would be much more compatible with the traditions of medicine than one which saw the doctor-patient encounter simply as a meeting of self-interested "providers" and "consumers" (a now-common language, which already displays the impact of market ideology). The notion of a "patient" could plausibly be maintained, something impossible with a purely economic model. At the historical core of the doctor-patient relationship has been the trust of patients that doctors act solely in their behalf. A market approach not only jeopardizes that trust, but supplants it with a commercial, contractual notion of human and professional relationships.

The Market as Behavioral Theory

To say that human beings act primarily out of self-interest is not, however, quite the same as to contend that it is possible to shape or influence their behavior by various economic incentives. The market idea, especially when used crudely, as a means of managing behavior, seems to me the last gasp of psychological behaviorism, going back to Watson, Skinner, and others: human behavior is the result of responses to behavioral stimuli, not significantly modified by conscious rationality. When market proponents propose the use of economic incentives and disincentives (e.g., copayments, deductibles, economic rewards or penalties for physicians) they work directly out of that tradition. It assumes that health-related behavior, including life and death themselves, can be given a price and that people will respond much as they would to the pricing of any other item. It is not so much that health is uniquely a commodity as it is that everything subject to pricing acts like a commodity. If financial incentives at the individual level of doctors and patients are a key instrument of market technique, competition among providers is the equivalent instrument at the health system level. Competition can reward efficiency, shape behavior, control costs, and forcefully focus institutional aims.

What seems clear, however, is that some of the techniques of the market can be detached from the larger scope of market theory and its interpretation of self-interested human nature. Thus even nonprofit organizations can well make use of market techniques such as competition among institutions and the use of financial incentives for particular types of behavior. The "internal markets" of the British National Health Service, put in place by the Thatcher government, provide another example of the use of market techniques in a governmental and nonprofit context.[15]

The Market as Political Theory and Ideology

The collapse of the Communist countries in the late 1980s gave the market a fresh impetus, advancing it not only as a superior way to manage national economies and institutions but also as embodying values of exceedingly useful political currency. Individualism as a value, established as the language of choice, autonomy, and self-determination by 1960s and 1970s liberals, turned out to be hardly less congenial to new conservatives. At the least, conservatives tied those values to a drive to reduce the power of government and, at the extreme, turned it into a radical moral as well as political libertarianism. In the eagerness to take advantage of the fall of Communism, it was only natural to posit a natural relationship between a free economy and a free society, each serving the other to the greater glory and strength of both. It is hardly any wonder, then, that the postsocialist nations have taken to the market as a vehicle for both economic and political recovery. A free economic market is seen as an ideological prerequisite for a free political society, a way of turning self-interest as a personal motivation into the national interest as a political motivation.

It is worth attending to the subtle relationship, too little noted in the medical context, between the liberal value of autonomy in private life and the market value of consumer choice in public economic life. For if liberals have characteristically been preoccupied, of late, with justice and equality (which they usually see as requiring an active role for government), the ultimate purpose of those goods is to allow individuals to choose their own way of life, with as little government interference as possible.

Here liberal and market-conservative ideas come together. It might well have been more difficult for the market to triumph ideologically had it not had the unwitting aid of earlier left-leaning liberalism, which gave a heavy weight to a morality of choice, was reluctant to judge the morality of the choices made, and strongly resisted overarching notions of the public interest or common good. As another economist, Donald Frey, has noted, in a passage that applies as well to some forms of liberal individualism as to the market ideology he is characterizing: "The notion of freedom [in the ethic of self-interest] is essentially without content, leaving each person 'free' to be a slave of the desires of the self. . . . The economic ethic poses the paradox that freedom emerges as the highest value in a system that is essentially a deterministic web of material incentives."[16]

Medicine, Health Care, and the Culture of the Market

If the market can be understood from these three different perspectives—as a theory of human nature, of behavioral change, and of political ideology—with at least one of them, behavioral theory, applicable in the nonprofit philanthropic sphere, it is nonetheless evident that the market is most persuasive when all three are joined together. This is exactly what seems to be happening in the marriage of medicine and the market. The market is being advanced as embodying a theory of human nature that coalesces well with a medicine oriented to helping individual people to be well and to enjoy a flourishing of their bodies. The market seems even more attractive when it is argued that the behavioral psychology of the market is just what is needed to control the high cost of medicine and its inefficient consumption. And then, to cap all that, medicine is better off yet when it can be joined with an ideology of choice, which is seen as a high patient value and necessary to preserve "consumers" from the ever-grasping tentacles of government bureaucracy or medical paternalism.

Seen in the best possible light, then, medicine and the market seem made for each other. What could be more self-interested than the desire for good health? What area of human activity—so infinite in its desires, so rife with inefficiency—could be more appropriate for the disciplinary behavioral incentives of the market than medicine? What part of human life could be a more fit candidate for the primacy of choice than what we do with our bodies and what is done with them? And what part of our lives should remain as intimate as the doctor-patient relationship, and thus be kept free of intrusive government?

These are strong claims, but some questions must be asked about them. Are they based on a compelling and historically sound understanding of the nature and goals of medicine? Is the ideology of the market appropriate to medicine? Is a market model of health care policy likely to best serve medicine and the health of populations?

How Well Can the Market Serve Medicine?

While it is surely true that our health is a matter of exceedingly important self-interest to us, it does not follow that medicine does, or should, take that self-interest as its starting point, even if individual patient welfare is the benchmark of the Hippocratic tradition. In a trivial sense, of course, medicine should start with patients' self-interest, for in questions of medicine and health care our lives can be at stake, without which nothing else much matters. More fundamentally, however, the historical good that medicine seeks is health, not autonomy or choice or the satisfaction of all human desires. And much that is required in the way of health can seem to thwart many interests other than life—particularly our desire on occasion to live badly regardless of the health consequences. While a market understanding of self-interest can surely accommodate a particular view of what constitutes genuine self-interest (the familiar "enlightened self-interest") as distinguished from apparent self-interest, this will only be true if the market is itself imbedded in a restraining culture. Many contemporary models of "the market" seem to embody purely instrumental and procedural notions of moral and social value.

A market notion of self-interest that reduces it to a right to make choices, indifferent to their content, is not compatible with the goals of medicine, however. A medicine that has become purely instrumental and empty of moral content in its practice would allow medical means to be used to serve whatever individuals took to be in their self-interest. But medicine works with a history, traditions, and values that have in view, implicitly but strongly, a substantive notion of individual and collective good, not reducible to an ideology of choice or the celebration of self-interest.[17] That good is health, the integrated well-being of mind and body. That good is not the same as choice, or autonomy, or the pursuit of self-interest.

There are reasons to doubt that an inherently instrumental theory of the market would serve medicine well. Part of the problem, however, in judging the claims of market proponents is that there does not now—and there may never—exist a perfect experimental model by which to test the market's claims of benefits to health care. There is no convincing evidence that the market will make medicine or health care systems more efficient, that competition will hold down costs, that economic incentives are the only ones that matter in medicine, or that the free play of the market will result in better individual or community health than any other way of organizing health care systems.

In many areas where the market has had more or less free play—the sale of automobiles, for example—costs have not been held down, competition has not been all that pure, and not all individual desires have been satisfied. In 1970, 38 percent of a young couple's annual income was needed to buy an automobile, whereas 50 percent was needed by the 1990s, hardly an advertisement for the power of the market to hold down costs.[18] Of course, the immediate objection is that in our world the market is rarely given a real chance—in this, the auto industry is no exception—and thus it has never effectively been tried. I understand this kind of response as nothing more than an expression of faith in the market, the kind of faith in an ideology that has all the markings of a secular-fundamentalist conviction about the way the world *ought* to work, and will work if just let alone. (I quickly add that the same has been true of socialist claims about the ideal way to achieve prosperity and equality in society. They are also professions of ideological faith, resting on weak empirical evidence.)

Both ideological capitalism and ideological socialism can find supportive evidence somewhere; neither is a total failure anywhere. But neither is well positioned to make the kinds of health-care-related claims that can once and for all settle their differences or establish the clear superiority of one. For just that reason claims about the efficacy of market values for med-

223

icine are likely never to find complete refutation *or* complete confirmation. Much will depend upon which values people prefer to seek, even if they don't attain them, and which liabilities they are willing to tolerate in the name of the ideological commitments they have made. Some people will give up many social goods if they get individual choice; others will give up individual choice for social goods (my own leaning).

A powerful objection to a market orientation in medicine has always been that it must inevitably lead to injustice, distributing goods in an impersonal and destructive way differentially to rich and poor. Money talks, as the saying goes, and a market economy in health care means that some can buy more than others, and some may not be able to afford any at all. China and Vietnam stand out as two countries that have moved sharply in a market direction, and at an enormous social and health cost to the poor.[19] The United States is the striking example of what happens when a nation refuses to guarantee basic minimum health care at an affordable price: millions of Americans have no health insurance at all, and millions of others have insecure insurance (which can be lost by, say, a job change) or inadequate insurance (not sufficient to cover a catastrophic illness). As if that example is not alarming enough, Allen Buchanan has shown how difficult, if not impossible, it will be for countries that now have universal health care to privatize their health care systems while maintaining equality of care; privatization contradicts that possibility by its very premises.[20]

Objections of this kind have always been recognized and, to varying degrees, acknowledged by market proponents. Most have granted that there must remain an important residual role for government to fill in the gaps that the market will create. But this acknowledgment creates an immediate dilemma: it concedes a necessary role to government, which must curtail a full working of the market to some degree, all the more urgently when the gap between rich and poor grows too great. In the process, market proponents also must concede that market dominance does not automatically guarantee a high level of average health, even if the health of some is fine. The United States not only fails to provide insurance coverage for some 15 percent of its population, it lags behind many other countries in infant mortality rates, average life expectancy, and other indices of health as well—and all the while its health care costs more per capita than any other system in the world.

Another objection to a market-dominated ideology is that, while it supports the idea of progress and technological innovation, there is no necessary correlation between the kind of innovation generated by the market and the kind of technology needed to improve overall health. On the contrary, innovative medical technology is designed to appeal to manufacturers' desire for profit and consumers' demands for constant medical improvements. Improved health may be a desired and foreseeable outcome, but profit is the initiating motive. An important reason for the rise of the technology- and outcome-assessment movement is the just lack of correlation between technological developments and health outcomes. Many technologies, though costly enough or desired enough to guarantee good profits to those who create and sell them, do not do what they are supposed to do, or do so in an excessively expensive way.

Does the market promote greater efficiency, control costs, and ensure quality in health care? That is one of the leading claims of its followers, but the evidence is mixed.[21] Competition is supposed to be one way of achieving efficiency, driving from the market those who cannot operate as efficiently as their competitors. But competition can also drive up costs, as happened in the 1970s and 1980s with hospital competition in the United States.[22] Competition requires matching the benefits offered by competitors, and thus sends all participants' costs spiraling upward together. The medical economist Burton A. Weisbrod has argued that not only may competition not optimize price, quantity, and quality, it may in fact be inefficient.[23]

As many others have noted, health care is different from

other commodities, and what may work in some industries may never work well in this one. Why? Patients ordinarily lack the necessary information to make good choices and, in any case, their employers will rarely offer them a full range of health care plans to choose from. "There is little evidence from the [United Kingdom] or elsewhere," the British economist Alan Maynard has written, "that competition in health care produces improvements in resource allocation."[24] As for the competitive possibilities of managed care, it has been noted that competition may lead not to greater efficiency but to competition for those people least likely to get sick.[25] At the same time, managed care faces the enormous challenge of maintaining quality in the face of competitive pressures to hold costs down.[26] Even so, competition has strong defenders; one of the least ideological, the philosopher Paul Menzel, believes that at least the problems of information and equity can be dealt with.[27]

A general claim of its proponents is that the market is a powerful engine for generating wealth and economic well-being. This is surely true in comparison with the abject failure of the Communist economies of postwar Central and Eastern Europe to improve the general standard of living. The argument for the market's power to generate wealth is double-edged, however. How can a system whose broad aim is the creation of wealth for all suddenly be expected to turn itself around and serve as a means of controlling costs (which are, after all, someone else's income)? To say that the market produces efficiency along with wealth will not do as an answer. Even efficient health care systems can be insupportably expensive. Efficiency of individual units in a health care system does not guarantee that the system as a whole will be affordable.

Intimate Relations

In the coming decades, medicine and health care systems will face two problems that will pose special difficulties for a market orientation. An aging population will cause one of the problems. How will a market-oriented medicine, intent on reducing the government burden of health care, find the social and moral resources necessary to put in place means of caring for the aged? In the twentieth century, governments were given the main responsibility for developing social security and health care programs for the elderly, though in the United States an important supplementary role was left for corporate pension plans and retiree health plans and for personal savings. At the end of the century, however, corporations are showing considerable reluctance to support expensive pension programs, whose demise is contributed to by the decline of union power. The employment trend in the United States, toward more low-paid hourly work and away from salaried employment, will create a larger and larger pool of people ill-prepared for a retirement also marked by weakened Social Security and government health care programs. The market is far better at meeting immediate short-term private interests than long-term collective interests, exactly the domain of health care for the elderly.

The other problem is in the sphere of intimate relations, where there will be growing pressure on young people to provide home care for their elderly parents. The strong trend in all countries to resist expanding nursing home and other custodial facilities for the elderly in favor of increased reliance on home and family care is likely to put extraordinary pressures on families, particularly on women, who are still often expected to be the primary caregivers in the home. There will be fewer family members at home to provide care, and there will surely be efforts by the affluent to buy the care they either cannot or do not want to provide. At the same time, a market medicine, if based solely on individual self-interest, will work against the bonds of family and intergenerational responsibility that must provide the moral motivation for informal home care.[28] That kind of care requires altruism and self-sacrifice. A moral model of solidarity, looking to mutual needs in the public and private spheres, will be far more helpful.

Competing Models of Health Care

I want now to place the market model among two other competing models of health care to identify its comparative strengths and weaknesses—the rights model and the solidarity model.

The *rights model* of health care, most vigorously pursued by political liberals over the past few decades, has typically taken as its starting point an argument that there is an individual right to health care and a corresponding right to equal access to health care.[29] Health is a basic human good and necessity, a critical ingredient of a right to life and thus the foundation of all other rights. The rights model thus rests on the health needs of the individual, not the collective good health of the community. A right to health care has no constitutional basis in the United States, nor has it been posited as a natural-law right. A considerable body of political and philosophical theory has, however, worked to develop a rights-based approach, using as its point of departure a claim to equal opportunity in society, facilitated by equal access to decent health care.[30]

At least that was the most powerful line of thought through the 1960s and 1970s. By the end of the 1970s, however, when efforts to develop some form of universal health care in the United States had stalled, there was a move—not always openly acknowledged—away from the explicit language of rights. Emphasis was instead placed on the obligation of government to provide decent access to health care for everyone. In the words of the 1983 Report of the President's Commission for the Study of Ethical Problems in Medicine and Biomedical and Behavioral Research, "Society has a moral obligation to ensure that everyone has access to adequate care without being subject to excessive burdens."[31] Yet in some ways this shift from the language of rights to that of government obligation was more rhetorical than substantive. To argue that the government has an obligation to provide some good is, logically, not different from a claim that an individual has a right to demand that good from government. But the shift in language does have the effect of softening what could otherwise appear to be an excessive, open-ended claim on community resources. That move helped address, though not fully or adequately, a serious problem with the individual-rights strategy: how and where to establish limits to the claims and how to compare, in times of resource shortage, the merits of competing rights claims. Most strikingly, by the time of the last major national health care reform effort, culminating (and collapsing) in 1994, proponents of universal care rarely used the language of rights.

The *solidarity* model of health care proceeds in a very different fashion. Sickness and death are understood to be shared threats to human life, a basic condition of human existence requiring a shared response. Human beings should understand their interdependence in the common need to struggle with disease and illness and respond to that need with solidarity. It is in both our individual and collective interest to band together, recognizing that we are all in the same general situation. The United States has always understood public education, fire fighting, police protection, and national defense as matters of common survival and solidarity in the face of shared needs and threats. But it has not extended the same thinking to health care, which has been left half in and half out of the market. A solidarity perspective has been the main foundation of European health care programs and the principal moral basis for making those programs universal. Even during the Margaret Thatcher and John Major years in the 1980s and 1990s, there was no thought in Britain of dismantling the popular National Health Service, a fully nationalized program run by government. Nor, even in the face of economic difficulties, has any other European country thought to eliminate basic health care, whether financed directly by government, by employer insurance, or by other mechanisms.

229

The concept of solidarity has been better able to deal with the problems of setting limits than a rights-based approach. It is taken for granted in Western Europe and Canada that the price of universal health care coverage entails some boundaries to that coverage, even if that fact is rarely spelled out openly. The fact that such systems are closed—with fixed budgets—also makes rationing easier. Yet the setting of limits, implicit or explicit, seems to have been more readily accepted in the immediate post–World War II decades than in more recent years. Countries that had managed to keep costs stable during the 1970s and 1980s, a time when they were increasing dramatically in the United States, found themselves under new pressures to increase their health care expenditures in the 1990s and facing greater public unwillingness (so it appears) to accept limitations on coverage. European trade unions, in particular, have resisted cutbacks in health care coverage (as have American unions). At the same time (hardly coincidentally) there was a waning of public willingness to let the welfare state grow and outbreaks of resistance to increased taxation. If, in the United States, the idea of a right to health care had to be softened in some way, the same became true of the idea of solidarity in Europe.

It may well be that, in the long run, a combined rights and solidarity approach would work best. The empathy and fellow-feeling that animate the idea of solidarity are also necessary to give the notion of a right to health care real bite. Rights will not be taken seriously if there is no feeling of empathy for those whose rights are at stake. For its part, the idea of solidarity could profit from the particularity of rights claims.

The *market* model of health care has yet to be fully defined. Few have proposed that health care be understood as a mere commodity, to be sold to those who can afford it and denied to those who cannot. No developed country has a pure market-model health care system. The more important issue has been to establish the relationship between market-oriented and government-oriented health care. I use the term "oriented" here to indicate a different weighting of emphasis, with the bias going toward either government or the market.

At one extreme, though with different shadings and gradations, would be the government-oriented programs of Western Europe. Because of economic pressures, as well as a strengthening of the ideological pull of the market, many of those programs are privatizing significant parts of their health care systems and, as in Great Britain's use of "internal markets," employing market techniques (particularly competition) to make their systems more efficient. While the notion of personal "choice" seems not to have the political force that it does in the United States, it also seems to be gathering some strength in European medicine, which has remained for the most part heavily paternalistic and authoritarian. Privatization has meant the development and official promotion of private-sector medicine, allowing an open market for the purchase of health care and for private medical practice independent of government-controlled medicine. Even Canadians, long resistant to private-sector medicine, are now debating whether to make a move in that direction. Privatization has also come to mean an increase in out-of-pocket expenditures, more deductibles, and greater difficulty in gaining access to a full range of government-provided services. Even so, in the European and Canadian context, government dominates the control of health care.

Near the other end of the continuum is the United States. Here the bias has been toward a market-oriented medicine, bringing government in primarily as a safety net. By historical accident, much health care in the United States is provided by private employers—though, since the costs of that care can be claimed as a business expense, there is an important, indirect government subsidy. With the collapse in 1994 of efforts to create a universal health care program in the United States, the momentum shifted back to a market emphasis, but with a special twist. The managed-care movement, ironically, captures many aspects of a universal health care program—centralized management, control of salaries and technology, limitation of patient and practitioner choice, for instance—but puts them into a market and competitive context. Competition is meant to be generated among those insurers and other sellers of managed care who want to gain the business of employers, state Medicaid programs for the poor, and the national Medicare program for the elderly. The purchase of many nonprofit hospitals and health care systems by for-profit enterprises has been a striking development, raising the possibility of a dominant for-profit medicine for the foreseeable future.

In theory, there is no reason why some combination of government and market programs cannot work out well enough. Everything will depend on where the balance is struck between the two orientations, and whether the reigning understanding of the market accepts the need for limits on it and for a strong, community-oriented set of complementary values.[32] As the case of the United States indicates, a weak commitment to government programs and a strong commitment to the market results in a system that is fine for most but terrible for a significant minority. The political and public willingness to tolerate large numbers of uninsured persons and to see a partial collapse of public health and community health programs is disturbing. There is nothing in the present managed-care or market emphasis to supply an antidote to that trend. Europeans and Canadians, while whittling away at the government orientation of their programs, seem, for the time being at least, sufficiently committed to a decent baseline of health care for all to withstand a crippling introduction of market techniques and goals.

Putting the Market to Work for Sustainability

I have contended that the most promising route to an economically sustainable medicine is a combination of improved public health programs and greater personal responsibility for maintaining health. Despite its theoretical attractions, the liability of this strategy is that the population bias of a public health emphasis seems too abstract to attract massive government funds, and the emphasis on personal behavior too concretely demanding to generate high hopes for its success. The present path, emphasizing high-technology rescue medicine, seems more congenial. But it is expensive, not cost-effective, and inherently unsustainable.

Can the market do better? The bet is that market methods can create incentives that will motivate individuals to control their personal health care costs, and motivate health care systems to manage aggregate costs better. This bet is unlikely to pay off. A market strategy, playing to individual desires, is more likely to stimulate new wants and demands than to dampen them. For every personal incentive to spend less money, there will be technological incentives to spend more: the attraction of new diagnostic possibilities for late-onset disease, coming out of recent genetic research; new rehabilitation options, coming out of computer and prosthetic advances; and new pharmaceutical choices, driven by an inventive, aggressive drug industry. Nothing in advanced capitalist technological societies seems to point toward less rather than more spending on technology. By contrast, the most insistent need of a sustainable medicine will be to dampen the use of technologies for marginal health care gains, working against medical perfectionism and risk-aversion. The market, however, is likely to see its greatest profits, and its greatest public lure, in just those technologies.

Far from accepting the need for a sustainable medicine, market proponents never argue for reduced medical consumption, for a limit on desires for improved health, for an acceptance of aging and death, or for some restraints on technological innovation. The optimistic assumption is that the market can economically support expansionary medical progress wherever it goes. But such optimism is no greater

233

than that which has undergirded pressure for a continuing, even expanded, government role: what the market would achieve by competition, government in the eyes of some would achieve by greater centralization, technology assessment, and more targeted research.

The main difference between these two competitive optimisms is that in Canada and Western Europe, government enthusiasts have had some decades to try out their ideas. Those ideas have proved to be increasingly unaffordable without more help than that provided by adding government cost-control techniques and regulation. The gradual move to a two-tier medicine throughout the developed world confirms that point: the market holds out its hand to provide the needed help. Market enthusiasts, however, can work with expectant hope, untested by much experience. The only available experience of any consequence comes from the American health care system, and though that experience appears to be anything but encouraging, American market proponents have been able to persuade would-be followers in other countries that the market has never really been given a fair chance here, being hobbled by government interference and poorly managed entitlement programs. This case has been made with particular effectiveness in Central Europe, where market thinking has become dominant. The outcome has yet to be evaluated. Whatever the available experience at present, however, there seems little reason to doubt that the market will have the momentum for the foreseeable future. Its ideas will be played out for better or worse, whether in the form of the massive privatization programs being pursued in Asia, Central Europe, and parts of Latin America, or in the more modified form being pursued in Great Britain, or in the introduction of two-tier health care in Western Europe, or in competitive managed care in the United States.

I have not painted an optimistic picture of the possibility of a good relationship between a sustainable medicine and the market. Their utterly dissimilar orientations provide in principle no solid reasons for doing so. Yet that general judgment must now be qualified by two considerations. The first is whether the medical market in the United States (or elsewhere, for that matter) can continue to be strongly influenced by an underlying moral culture that will soften some of its potential sharp edges and humanize its aspirations. The second consideration is whether some features of market thinking can be usefully adopted without accepting the entire market ideology.

1. *The Market and Its Cultural Context.* As noted earlier in this chapter, Adam Smith's market was by no means an amoral, impersonal force, but rather part of a cultural context that would influence and modify it. In the American context things have often worked out just that way: witness the repudiation of the unregulated robber-baron capitalism that marked the late nineteenth and early twentieth centuries, the willingness of many employers over the decades to provide job security and benefits beyond what a strict devotion to profits might have dictated, and both federal and state willingness to regulate the nastier workings of the marketplace, limiting what can be done in the name of profit. The rapidity with which many states, and Congress, have intervened to control for-profit medicine and managed care—as with the length of hospitalization after childbirth—is testimony that the tradition (for so it might be called) endures.

Hardly less important will be the extent to which for-profit, market-dominated medicine is managed by people with a strong sense of civic responsibility. No one expects a for-profit organization to conduct itself like a public charity. It would soon go under and its managers would be dismissed. At the other extreme, the notion of "tough" managers—indifferent to the human costs of what they do, focused only on the bottom line—finds a mixed reception in the United States. The recent public and political reaction against insensitive "downsizing" is one sign of this ambivalence. While there is no clear picture of just what the ideal manager should be like, there seems at least a general expectation that a manager must balance the needs of the community and employees against the return owed to stockholders. The open question at the moment is the extent to which this expectation will become and remain a part of for-profit American medicine, particularly in managed-care organizations. Jerome P. Kassirer, editor-in-chief of *The New England Journal of Medicine,* spoke for many doctors when he wrote: "Market-driven health care creates conflicts that threaten our professionalism . . . increasingly physicians will be forced to choose between the best interests of their patients and their own self-interest."[33] Will this happen to a great extent? The answer is uncertain. Competitive pressure, on the one hand—which in part dictates that managed-care organizations appear humane and sensitive to the needs of their clients—and political pressure, on the other, to behave well push in the direction of humaneness.

What remains to be seen is whether a softened, humane working of the market can be maintained. As competition becomes much tougher, the economic pressures to cut costs become still stronger. A larger and larger portion of the health care industry is profit-oriented. American business has a poor reputation for thinking about the long term, a mixed record in taking account of moral and social values, and comparatively little experience until recently in trying to manage large health care systems. Much, therefore, remains uncertain.

A medical market that moved in the direction of the Chicago school, with its reduction of all behavior to economic behavior and the ruthlessness and hard-heartedness that can inspire, would be a menace to sustainability. The bottom line would be king, fed by a no-holds-barred effort to make as much money as possible regardless of the social consequences. Yet whether it will be possible for the medical market to produce humane, high-quality medical care remains an open question. It is not impossible by any means, but neither it is assured.

2. Using the Market Wisely. Where the market does have something useful to say is in its recognition of the uses of financial incentives and disincentives. This is a delicate matter. There is no doubt that behavior can be changed by such incentives. Yet overharsh incentives can threaten not only medical equity but also the possibility of medical morality.[34] A purely market solution to the delivery of health care, forcing people to pay wholly out of their own pockets, would do considerable harm to large numbers of people who could not afford to pay. That point is so obvious that the pure market approach has few proponents. At the other extreme, if there are no financial constraints whatever on individual desires for health care, or on the meeting of all needs however marginal, then there can be no possibility of controlling costs.

The problem, then, comes down to this: can financial incentives and disincentives be sufficiently well orchestrated, and sufficiently nuanced, to accomplish three goals? The first goal is to firmly and effectively restrain marginal demand for health care by making people think twice about whether to insist on care they might otherwise desire. The second is to ensure that such financial pressure would not significantly hurt most people's health. It might increase risk to some extent— for a greater acceptance of risk is a key element of a sustainable medicine—but not enough to pose serious statistical hazards to the health of most of us. The third goal is for the incentives not to threaten equitable access to care in any significant way. If those three goals could be met, then the stronger emphasis I have proposed for individual responsibility could have the additional support of financial incentives. Money incentives could both encourage people to take good care of themselves in order to avoid medical needs as much as possible in the first place, and then discourage them from too quickly turning to medicine to meet such needs once they arise.

I will not attempt to propose here some specific mechanisms for doing that, but it is well known that copayments for treatment, even small ones, reduce demand, as does imposing a deductible before full support kicks in. Financial benefits or rewards for those who improve their health status, or eliminate unhealthy behavior, can be effective too. Financial penalties for those who fail to do what they need to do are reasonable as well. There is nothing, in short, particularly mysterious about the kinds of financial incentives that will decrease the demand for health services.

It is more difficult to avoid increasing risks to health and threatening equitable access. The only way to avoid the former possibility is by analyzing the evidence (which needs to be better collected) concerning the impact of incentives on health status and medical risk. Inevitably, equitable access will be compromised to some extent by financial incentives and penalties. These will be irrelevant to people who have enough money to be indifferent to costs, and they will be taken more seriously by those with less money. Equitable access does not, however, require *absolutely* identical access and a level financial field; that is impossible to achieve in any case. The rich always do better than everyone else. The more important issue is whether any discrepancies open up excessive gaps between the rich and poor, with the health status of the poor far more threatened by financial incentives and disincentives than the health status of the rich. That should not be allowed to happen, and need not happen if there is a systematic effort to monitor the gaps that exist and to keep them as small as possible.

In much the same vein, if it could be shown that competition among health care providers delivered more efficient services with no decline in quality, then that market mechanism could be acceptable enough and could conceivably contribute to a sustainable medicine. My own guess is that that will never happen, in great part because it will be exceedingly difficult to create effective competitive markets in health care. It will be no less hard to use competition to dampen the cost-increasing impact of an ongoing commitment to medical progress and technological innovation. To the extent that these remain strong values, health care costs will be driven up. If some organizations arise, however, that offer steady-state medicine, do not pretend to be keeping up with the technological Joneses, and focus their efforts on good programs of disease prevention and primary care, they might most effectively compete for patients. And if there are strong financial incentives to join such organizations—because their costs are strikingly lower—they could draw a large group of people.

If one thinks of "the market" not as a package that must be taken whole or not at all, but rather as offering a variety of values and strategies, then it could be helpful. A wholehearted turn to the market must remain the main threat to a population-based sustainable medicine. Used carefully, with an eye to health outcomes and the need for equity, the market has some valuable possibilities. That much said, it remains unclear to me whether a discriminating use of market mechanisms is possible. In theory, yes; in practice, who knows? There is nothing deterministic about all this. We can get the kind of use of the market we, as a political society, want, if we want it seriously enough and use sufficient political and moral force to bring it about. James Q. Wilson, speaking in a way that reflects the Adam Smith tradition, has put the matter nicely: "The problem for capitalists is to recognize that, while free markets will ruthlessly eliminate inefficient firms, the moral sentiments of man will only gradually and uncertainly penalize immoral ones. But, while the quick destruction of inefficient corporations threatens only individual firms, the slow anger at immoral ones threatens capitalism—and thus freedom—itself."[35] This statement could usefully be posted in the boardroom of every for-profit health care organization, from the pharmaceutical industry to managed-care companies. Some have already heeded the message, but others have not.

CHAPTER EIGHT

Equity and a Steady-State Medicine

"Life is unfair." John F. Kennedy said that, but any doctor could say the same. Illness and disease visit people in unjust, unequal, and unforgiving ways. Medicine has sought to combat that unfairness by going after the causes and manifestations of illness. National health care systems have sought to engage the resources of government in that struggle, doing what they can to put medical skills within the economic grasp of their citizens. While there have been fierce political battles about how best to do so, every government espouses the principle of decent access to health care. Even unrepentant libertarians who would do away with a government role altogether argue that an unfettered free market is the best way to achieve equity: give everyone an equally free choice to choose the kind and degree of health care they want.

I do not here want to enter into the argument about

which kind of health care system is most likely to achieve equitable access to health care (though I believe a single-payer system would do the best job). Instead, I want to establish a prior point: that equitable health care systems in the future will only be possible with a sustainable, steady-state medicine. An inherently expansionary, progress-obsessed medicine cannot fail to generate inequity in the distribution of its benefits.

The goal of equitable health care is to allow all people decent access to affordable and efficacious care. The moral motivation for that goal ought to be a shared sense of empathy in the community, a common perception that the burdens of illness and disability can befall everyone, and indirectly affect everyone, and thus should be commonly shouldered. What would count as equitable access to health care?[1] I want to define it not in individual terms but in terms of population access to health care. Equitable access can thus be defined as the availability of affordable health care to a population as a whole, where all citizens have a (1) statistically good chance of receiving, over their lifetime, the kind of health care they need to (2) reduce the likelihood of premature death and of physical and mental disability.

Notice that I do not include in this definition a focus on meeting each individual need and desire. The emphasis falls instead on improving the odds of good health for a population as a whole, and on reducing the statistical chance that any given individual will fall ill. The available health care will be organized in accordance with an effort to determine the most statistically likely causes of premature death and disability. The available diagnostic and therapeutic strategies will be oriented to providing the care most likely to be useful and effective. Two clear implications follow from this definition: some people, those with statistically uncommon conditions, will not fare well in this health care system—there will be orphan diseases and orphan patients; and, when patients are under treatment, they will be provided only with the kind of care statistically likely to help most, but not all, of them.

This may seem like a harsh definition of equitable access, and it surely has some features that put it in that light. But it has three principal purposes designed to enhance, not diminish, the probability of better health for more people. First, it is meant to help ensure that excessive sums are not spent on medical care; instead, it emphasizes the provision of that kind of health care which improves the health of populations as a whole. It is thus meant to take serious account of the persuasive contention of Robert G. Evans and others that a country can provide too much medical care and that such care can be a threat to good health.[2] It could also help stimulate the spending of money on other aspects of society that have an important indirect role in improving health, such as education and employment.

Second, by focusing on population rather than individual health, my definition of equitable access is meant to curtail medical care at the margins—meaning both statistically uncommon medical conditions, and treatments that aim for statistically unlikely outcomes. Here the aim is to work against the excessive emphasis upon individual risk elimination and medical perfectionism so largely responsible for many of medicine's economic problems.

Third, this strategy is meant to stimulate a great personal responsibility for health by serving notice that expensive marginal treatments, particularly the high-technology kind, will not be provided to enhance individual outcomes. This would also discourage the development and dissemination of expensive technologies with marginal statistical benefits for population health.

In seeking an equitable medicine it is the gross inequities, not all inequities, that must be targeted. What are those gross inequities? The most obvious are racial and economic discrepancies in life expectancy (particularly disastrous for black males), as well as in infant mortality rates and prenatal care. Poverty is a major source of inequity, showing up in the gap between poor and nonpoor in vaccination rates, in screening for breast cancer and other illnesses, and in physician contacts more generally. The fact that 41 million people in the United States are uninsured is itself a grave inequity.[3] On a worldwide scale, the gap in almost every health category between the rich and poor countries, but most strikingly in life expectancies and infant mortality rates, is a more massive form of inequity. Unless a sustainable medicine is developed, the chances of closing that gap are diminishingly small.[4]

Five Tensions

I want now to rework five themes of this book with respect to their implications for equitable health care. I will state them in terms of some basic tensions, each of which can be resolved in a nonsustainable, technological direction. I want to show that, if the resolution is pressed, instead, in the sustainable direction I have been advocating, the possibility of an equitable medicine is greatly enhanced. I use the word "enhanced" deliberately. There is far more to creating an equitable health care system than starting with some helpful values and predispositions. I only want to argue that the reigning values of contemporary medicine in our era have demonstrably made equity harder to achieve and maintain. After I have laid out the five tensions, I want to apply my general line of thinking to the provision of medical care at different stages in the life cycle (hoping to illustrate along the way the value of a life-cycle perspective), and then to propose an approach to a basic benefits package that would incorporate the elements I have earlier developed.

The tensions I want to discuss are those between manipulating nature and respecting nature; pursuing health and accepting illness; promoting public obligation and accepting personal responsibility; seeking personal choice and tolerating imposed limits; and chasing progress and living with a steady-state medicine.

243

1. *Manipulating Nature and Respecting Nature.* The need to manipulate nature, to bend it to our will, has some obvious roots in our own human nature. We are smart enough to understand that nature is not always friendly, that it can sicken and maim and cripple and kill us, and sometimes all of those together, all at once, or little by little. This is the scene that modern medicine contemplated some time ago, putting to one side the older view that our body can take care of itself if properly respected and handled with care. Medicine went on the attack, seeking through research to find the causes of disease and through technological diagnosis and therapy to rid us of those causes and relieve us of their symptoms. Even as it found ways to benefit almost everyone, it also opened the way to eventual inequity. Partly this was inadvertent: some conditions (e.g., heart disease) proved more amenable to a technological solution than others (e.g., Alzheimer's). But some of the inequity resulted from deliberate actions: special targets were chosen because of their profit potential, as in the case of the search for anticlotting agents to combat heart attacks.

Despite much success in struggling against it, nature has not let us off easily. It has struck back by making our latter-day advances against it increasingly difficult. It will not give up the territory of aging populations so cheaply as it did the territory of infant mortality. It has given us, of late, an increased life expectancy often overshadowed by frailty and chronic disease.

Nature has also reminded us, however, that if we live reasonably sensible lives—not smoking; watching our diet; exercising; getting enough sleep, for instance—we have a far better than even chance of living a long life even without the intervention of medicine. It has no less reminded us that it is not nature alone that causes us problems, but the way nature interacts with the environment humans have created. Nature often reminds us that the body has immense capacities for self-renewal and self-healing, that its resiliency in the face of insult is formidable.

In developed societies, a steady-state medicine will keep

the difficulties and obstacles of advanced progress clearly before its eye. The reality of those difficulties, not the progress-driven, anxiety-dependent hope that research will overcome them, would be the reigning image: Warning—be careful about your scientific dreams. A steady-state medicine will not seek cure and disease amelioration first in technology, because (from the historical record) it will expect that approach to add expense as rapidly as improvement. Instead, it will go first with the evidence that public health and good primary care are the proven strategies for population health, and that, if technology must be used to respond to the inevitable failure of public health in some or many individual cases, the only valuable technologies are those that have been shown *in advance* to offer cost-effective diagnosis and efficacious treatment—that is, a clear benefit.

Of course, the idea of "clear benefit" is ambiguous. I stipulate a clear benefit as one where over 50 percent of patients will show a significant improvement in their medical condition, and where the costs of even that improvement are not excessive in the context of competing medical needs and possible alternative expenditures. The 50 percent standard is high, but only such a high standard is compatible with a sustainable medicine. It should apply to both diagnostic and therapeutic technologies. To be sure, so rigorous a standard will, predictably, lead to the harm or death of some portion of the population at risk. A sustainable medicine can do no other than accept this unpleasant reality; and it should not shirk admitting that fact openly.

A steady-state medicine will do nothing *deliberately* to extend the present average life expectancy in developed countries. Nor will it carry out research to save low-birthweight babies beyond present limits (450 to 500 grams), or to find the cure of every disease, or to eradicate every last case of those diseases generally under control, or to find ways to extend the last months of those suffering from ordinarily fatal disease. It is precisely those efforts that threaten equity. While the developing countries should work to achieve health parity with the developed countries—in quality of care as well as equitable access—they should also found their systems on a base of public health and primary care, adding only those technologies that have demonstrated clear benefit. That way they can raise the general level of health without unfairly skewing it in favor of some groups of patients over others.

Nature has been brought to heel, not fully but enough to make it easier to live with if we pay attention to its cautionary messages. We can only expect unending economic and social trouble if we try to push nature much further. We will be courting increased inequity. It is time to declare a truce and to enjoy what we now know, in a way that can be available to all.

2. *Pursuing Health and Accepting Illness.* As René Dubos reminded us some years ago, perfect health is a mirage.[5] It is no less a mirage to believe that equality in medical outcome—perfect health for *all*—is possible. The mirage shimmers because it basks in the sun of scientific optimism and often-desperate hope. Nonetheless, since none of us cares to be sick, much less to be stricken and die, we will and must pursue health, individually and collectively. Good health is as much a social need as an individual one. Fortunately, most people in the developed countries enjoy reasonably good health: they survive their childhood, rarely get sick as adults, and face serious illness only as they grow old. Not all people, of course, are lucky, even those who live well—which is why the costs of most health care systems are incurred by a comparatively small proportion of the citizens, ordinarily between 10 and 15 percent of them. Even so, for most of us living in developed countries, and now even in many developing countries, if childhood (and, for women, childbirth) can be safely negotiated there is a far better than even chance of growing old. Old age is now the fate of most of us.

Technological medicine is turned to, however, because it

seems to speak best to individual health needs. What I need for my health may not be what you need for yours. While an X ray may pick up my lung cancer, it may take an MRI to pick up your brain tumor. While a simple family history may determine the risk of my children for Tay-Sachs disease, it may take a complex genetic screen to determine the susceptibility of yours to early-onset Alzheimer's. While a less fatty diet may reduce my risk of death from heart disease, your unavoidable genetic risk may require complicated coronary bypass surgery. So it goes, and so it is that technology will always be looked to as a way of preserving or promoting our personal, individual health, or helping us to get through a life marked by poor health. But this very process of homing in on our individual needs in the name of equality of individual outcome has served to generate inequity.

A steady-state medicine will, however, stress that a monomaniacal push to improve individual health can utterly destroy the possibility of an equitable and sustainable medicine—and possibly, through anxiety and socially approved hypochondria, personal lives as well. Health is a good, but always a temporary good. The cure of one disease in a person will inevitably and invariably be followed by another disease. Nature is bountiful in producing successor maladies for those that have been cured, whether in populations or individuals. This means that equality of outcomes will forever remain elusive, and a health care system that too strenuously pursues that goal in the name of equity will find economic stability elusive as well.

A steady-state medicine will have to do that which doctors personally most hate to do, and which medicine in general has most steadily resisted: it will have to make clear to people that they will die. Hippocrates did not want to say that. The medicine I want to promote will not pretend that if patients get over their cancer they are home free; or that if cancer is cured, average life expectancy will dramatically improve; or that an end to heart disease is an end to death; or that a cure for Alzheimer's disease is just a matter of time and research

247

money. "Americans," the Nobel laureate Francis Crick noted, "have a peculiar illusion that life is a disease which has to be cured. . . . Everyone gets unpleasant diseases and everyone dies at one time. I guess they are trying to make life safe for senility."[6]

A steady-state medicine will work to convince people—through persuasion if possible, and through their pocketbook if necessary—that they must accept the finitude of the body, the fragility of the mind, and the fleeting nature of health. A little fatalism, a little loosening up in the search for health, a little acceptance even of that nature red in tooth and claw seem necessary here. They will make equity more possible. The setting of bounds to aspiration is a necessary constituent of equity (and explains why the Western European health care systems were so successful for so long).

3. *Promoting Public Obligation and Accepting Personal Responsibility.* What do we owe our fellow citizens when they become sick? What ought we to expect from others when we become sick? We all face the threat of illness and death and know that we need the assistance of other people to increase our chances of overcoming them. The idea of solidarity thus seems the right one on which to found a health care system, underscoring as it does our common plight and common need for assistance. Empathy and a lively sense of dependence undergird solidarity as a social value. Universal health care, lacking in the United States but taken for granted in other developed countries, is the proper expression of solidarity, taking everyone in and leaving no one out. The equality of fundamental need, though variably expressed, is the basis for an equitable health care system.

It is far easier to make the case for public health and population benefits as an expression of solidarity and equality than it is to make the case for advanced technology useful to individuals. It is not that individuals do not count; far from it. It is just that a properly oriented health care system must take as its point of departure what it can do to benefit all and what it does most efficiently. The pursuit of individual benefit is a bottomless financial pit, particularly when "benefit" constantly changes because of technological innovation. If health care is to be extended to most, if not all, individual needs, it is perfectly appropriate to expect our fellow citizens to take as much responsibility for their own health as possible. If they want us to think about their special needs, they in turn have to ask what they can reasonably do to minimize those needs. This does not mean we should reject caring for them if they fail to take responsibility—as many surely will—but it does mean that we will work hard to urge, even force, them to minimize their health risks. There needs to be a sharing of responsibility to parallel an equity of access and assistance.

Every health care system now requires some thoughtful and publicly articulated priorities, even though the idea of priority-setting is itself controversial. At the top of my list will be palliative care for those who are going to die, public health and primary care of benefit to populations; at the bottom, high-technology medicine of benefit to individuals. But if health care systems are to continue being able to afford to get to the bottom of that list, there will have to be a reduction in demand for those technological services. That can be brought about by the usual methods of cost containment, but those will not work well unless people have tried to keep themselves well enough to reduce the need in the first place. That is the equality of responsibility.

A steady-state, equitable medicine will therefore both guarantee a decent basic level of health care for all, and at the same time expect personal responsibility from all in return. It will make use of the market when the market is an effective way of controlling costs, but it will never let the market become the dominant model for providing health care. The market cannot guarantee a basic floor of care, and is always liable to increase the disparity in available care. Nonetheless, market techniques are useful for encouraging personal responsibility

nd (if employed with caution) for penalizing those who fail to
exercise it.

4. *Seeking Personal Choice and Tolerating Imposed Limits.*
The desire to choose one's physician and to have significant
control over one's treatment has marked medicine in the developed countries. While there is a fair degree of disparity in
the control given to patients in their treatment, most health
care systems have worked to allow a choice of physicians.
More generally, all health care systems have seen an increase
in patient demands, fueled in part by medical advances and
in part by patients' greater knowledge of medical options and
possibilities. Yet, interestingly, no data that I have been able to
discover show any correlation between patient choice of physician and health outcomes. Nor is there any evidence that patient choice of treatment significantly affects outcomes either,
however much it may satisfy patient desires.

Yet a focus on outcomes alone probably does not address
the motives behind the desire for choice. Patients want to
choose their physician because they seek someone with whom
they can emotionally connect, with whom they feel at ease,
and whom they can trust to give them full attention. Since
anxiety and insecurity are a significant part of the suffering of
illness, particularly serious illness, it is comforting and reassur-
ing to have a physician whom one can trust. Moreover, where
choice among treatments is possible, exercising it can give a
patient a greater sense of control over her destiny.

The obvious problem is that both kinds of choice cost
money. Nothing, in principle, works against equity so much
s a patient seeing his suffering, or that of his family, as more
nportant than the suffering of others, and a doctor who be-
ves her obligations are solely to her patients *individually*,
ose benefit she is obliged to seek above all else. Cost con-
, and a prudent use of resources, will require a limit on
ice. The limits may be on the treatments that physicians
use, or for which insurance coverage may be provided,

or on the availability of some treatments at all. The aim will be a "more efficient use of an existing level of resources."[7] When to those limits are added restrictions on what patients may choose, or choose only at the cost of high copayments or deductibles, then the limitations may be severe indeed. Just how severe will be a function of the resources available to the health care system.

A steady-state, equitable medicine will have to limit, not expand, patient choice. It will require frank rationing.[8] It will work to resist patient demands, particularly demands stimulated by market pressure and incentives. It will also work to resist the medicalization of social and personal problems, which obviously increases the demands on medicine. At the same time, it will where possible try to give patients their choice of primary care physicians, but always with the understanding that one of the duties of those physicians is to help control the costs of health care, mainly by working within agreed-upon boundaries. Managed care is on the right track here. A sustainable, equitable medicine is not compatible with maximum choice, but it may be compatible with enough choice to allow patients needed comfort and security in their caretakers.

5. Chasing Progress and Living with a Steady-State Medicine. One of modern medicine's greatest claims to glory is the progress it has made in understanding and treating disease. Belief in progress, and its endless pursuit, are at the heart of contemporary medical values. Sustainability as a goal, by contrast, presumes that constant change and progress must be resisted because they tend to produce a medicine that is economically and psychologically unsustainable. A progress-dominated perspective is also a great hazard to equity, since there is no way to ensure that the progress will be socially affordable or that its fruits will benefit the population as a whole; the latter is as unlikely as the former.

A steady-state, equitable medicine will treat the idea of

unlimited progress as a major obstacle. It will understand the desire for progress, as well as its considerable future possibilities—we hurt and get sick, and something can be done about that. But a steady-state medicine will work against the confident notion that all progress is affordable, that all progress brings real benefit and increased equality of outcome, and that there is a moral duty to pursue progress. The escalating costs of all health care systems show the limits of affordability. They equally show the deleterious impact on equitable care as more governments back away from their earlier dedication to equitable access for all. While there may be a moral duty to help people in general live long and healthy lives, there can be no obligation to pursue unlimited progress. Illness and death remain natural human conditions, and there can be no duty utterly to root them out. That is a fool's mission.

The market will be the greatest promoter of progress and innovation, for only thus can it continue to generate growth in profits. And I want to stress that individuals should always be free to buy what they want on the medical market. But the institutions that pay for health care—governments, businesses, or insurance companies—should understand that they are not required to meet each and every need, or to respond to each and every market innovation. The goal for those who provide care should be decent care, not up-to-the-minute, state-of-the-art care. Precisely that latter goal, now usually imposed by public pressure, is the most serious threat to equity. It must be changed. A steady-state medicine will be a "good enough" medicine, not the best conceivable medicine. But it will be available to all. A sustainable medicine can be nothing other than that.

Living with and Within the Life Cycle

I have contended throughout this book that medicine should root itself in the life cycle, aiming to get people through a full and long life. The average life expectancies now achieved in the developed countries are sufficient to constitute that "full and long life." Any future increases in average life expectancy (which there surely will be) should be encouraged to come about *only* as the natural by-product of healthier lifestyles and the consequent reduction of illness in old age, not as the result of deliberate efforts. The main focus of a sustainable and steady-state medicine will be to improve the quality of life—by which I mean to reduce the risk of sickness and disability—within a limited life cycle. A basis for equity can thus be established by virtue of that limit. What kinds of goals should then be sought within that life cycle to achieve such an aim? I will sketch an imaginative picture of the future, not seeking to be definitive but choosing just a few sample issues where a steady-state medicine will create a different set of practices, attitudes, and expectations.

1. Procreation, Birth, and Childhood. Some couples who want children are infertile and turn to medicine to help them have a child. How far should medicine go in seeking to reduce infertility? Not far. While the inability to have a child does represent the failure of an ordinary biological capacity, and can be a great psychological loss for a couple, there is no societal need for increased fertility and much to argue against it. Nonetheless, given the pain felt by infertile couples, some resources should be made available to help them, and some research aimed at the most common causes of infertility should go forward, though with a low priority.

Health care plans that do not provide automatic coverage for infertility relief are perfectly appropriate. Fertility treatments are expensive and not very successful. In vitro fertilization, for instance, helps no more than 20 to 25 percent of those who turn to it, and then only at a few centers. When treatment for infertility is provided it should be limited. Some couples will then never be able to have the children they want. That is a genuine shame, but there is no need or obligation for medicine to help each and every couple have a child. A steady-state medicine will accept a relatively high rate of infertility; to reduce infertility, it will depend more on public health measures than on the more complex and often highly expensive technologies now employed. Public health measures would include intensified efforts to reduce sexually transmitted disease and education to better inform women of the decreased fertility caused by delayed procreation.

If a steady-state medicine will feel no compulsion to rid the world of infertility, it will feel even less obligation to use genetic or other techniques to give couples the kind of children they want. Apart from helping couples, through genetic counseling and prenatal diagnosis, to avoid the most damaging kinds of abnormalities in their children, medicine will not lend itself to the enterprise of perfect babies, much less parent-designed children. Nor will it even try to guarantee that all parents will have healthy children, though it will seek to improve outcomes where that can be done at a reasonable cost and use of medical resources. No parent should be so unfortunate as to have *two* handicapped children, and a special effort should be made to help those for whom that is a distinct probability. But it is the sheerest medical perfectionism to seek as a goal that no parent should have even one such child.

Most couples will, with proper prenatal care, have a healthy child. The odds are entirely in their favor. A sustainable medicine will accept the fact that some small minority will not have a healthy child, and it will not struggle against that sad fact. An excess zeal for biological equality will undermine overall equity. Some children will be born at a dangerously low birthweight or with severe medical problems. A steady-state medicine will limit the resources it makes available to save every such child, just as it will limit funding for research to improve outcomes. Babies as small as 450 to 500 grams can now be saved, though often their outcomes are poor. It would be reasonable to attempt to improve those outcomes, but unreasonable to seek to save still-smaller babies.

The biological difficulty of coping with inadequate lung development should be taken as a signal that a natural boundary has been met, which medicine has no obligation to cross. Sustainable medicine will, moreover, seek to limit efforts to salvage every child born with serious and particularly multiple handicaps. It will do what it can within the limits of a moderate technological effort, but it will avoid lengthy technological struggles; there will be a bias against them.

2. *Flourishing in Adulthood.* A steady-state medicine will work to avert premature death and a life of mental or physical disability. Breast cancer in women under sixty-five is an obvious research target, but so are many other lethal conditions. For victims of accidents and stroke, rehabilitation will be important, and there is considerable room for research in this field. But health promotion and disease prevention programs directed against strokes and accidents will receive significantly heightened attention in a steady-state medicine. Two points will be made clear to the public. One of them is that the living of a healthy life will have its own rewards, in a reduced chance of illness, disability, and premature death. The other will be a tougher message: high-technology rescue medicine will be scarce for the elderly, limited for babies and children, and reduced for all other age groups.

It will be in the care of adults (roughly, people between twenty-one and sixty-five years old) that technological medicine will be most prominently and justifiably used, even in a steady-state medicine that seeks to limit it.[9] The healthiest possible living habits cannot guarantee perfect health or safety from accidents or infections. Yet since a steady-state medicine will work to limit health care budgets—aiming in some countries to spend more per capita than at present, and in others (notably the United States) less—it will not attempt to meet every need or avoid every risk but will set priorities for working within a limited budget.

Expensive medical screening, whether for individuals or

for populations, is particularly open to skepticism. Screening for low-risk cancer probabilities, or heart disease, or other conditions, should be limited, done only when strong evidence exists of a significant benefit for many, not a few. Medical perfectionism will again be understood as the special enemy, whether in pursuing unlikely cures (as in some forms of cancer therapy) or in overusing diagnostic strategies to rule out all possibility of untoward or low-probability hazards or missed diagnoses. The routine screening of women under fifty for breast cancer is an example. Some cancers will thereby be missed. That's not perfect, but it's good enough. Not every elderly male needs to be pressured into prostate cancer screening, even though it could benefit some. That's not perfect, but it's good enough.

3. *Aging.* Once people have made it past the point of a premature death (a point I would set in the range of sixty-five to seventy years), then the highest priority for medicine should become not to avert death but to enable people to live as comfortable and secure a life as possible. High-technology medicine ought surely to be made available, but the government's obligation to provide that kind of medicine to people in, say, their late seventies or early eighties should be limited, even excluded or severely limited in the case of expensive technologies. The possibility that health care systems will go bankrupt after the turn of the twenty-first century is evident in the demographic and financial projections. Those who want to receive expensive forms of health care well into old age should be expected to pay for them out of their own pockets, or to pay a particularly high deductible or copayment.

The important point is a lively recognition that, with aging populations and constantly developing technologies, the greatest future threat to a steady-state medicine will be the costs of health care for the elderly.[10] Those costs are the principal threat to equity between the young and the old in the years ahead—one group, in effect, running away with the health care budget. Even now the elderly are a major factor in the escalation of health care costs worldwide. Unless that can be controlled, there is no hope for a sustainable medicine. The aging of the population cannot be stopped; only the technologies and intensified services that can be used to extend or improve their lives can be halted. They should be.

However, even as it worked to set technological limits — and used age as an important criterion for doing so — a sustainable medicine should work to ensure decent economic support for the elderly. This would include good long-term and home care, and of course adequate low-cost primary care medicine throughout their lives. That level of care may be all we can afford after 2010 or so, and even it will pose problems (with the costs of long-term care for those over eighty ordinarily exceeding those of acute-care medicine). That is all the more reason for it to be understood that both unlimited beneficial acute-care medicine and unlimited beneficial care of other kinds will be impossible in the future. There is no reason to believe, however, that such limitations will produce any decline in the general health status and life expectancy of the elderly, heavily dependent as both are on earlier health habits and other factors. At worst, potential improvements in the health of the elderly might come more slowly in the future.

4. *Dying.* Perhaps only in the United States is there active interest in, and worry about, the high cost of dying and excessive efforts to prolong life. In this country some 30 percent of the health care costs of the elderly come in the last year of life.[11] But the cost of dying is likely to become a greater concern everywhere, since it is a function of the availability of technologies that can marginally extend life, and a manifestation of patient demand. It may sound paradoxical to say that patient demand is a driving force behind the supposed excessive end-of-life treatment, but I believe this to be true. Patients in general say that they do not want excessive treatment, or to have their dying prolonged. But when the time for dying

comes, they are perfectly capable of matching their doctors in their desire to see if just a *little* bit more might be done to gain a little more life. The seduction of a technological death is that it *may* provide one more chance at life. Since there is usually some small (even if vanishingly small) possibility of doing so, that chance is often embraced, even if it contradicts earlier statements about a desire not to have such treatment.[12]

A sustainable medicine will accept death in old age as a natural and inevitable part of life. Particularly because it will be encouraging lifestyles that enhance the possibility of a minimal degree of sickness and disability prior to advanced old age, it will be especially concerned not to lose the economic advantage of those gains to excessive technology at the end of life. With the elderly, it will have established limits on expensive life-extending technologies in order to avoid the subversion of gains in the compression of morbidity. With other patients, it will establish clear criteria of likely treatment efficacy before allowing such treatment to proceed.

A steady-state medicine will educate its physicians to understand that the care of the dying is as much their responsibility as the care of those who can be cured. It will understand that medicine works within the boundaries of the life cycle, and that it must worry as much about how people are treated at the end of that cycle, when they are soon to leave it, as about how they are treated at its beginning and in its middle. Steady-state medicine will seek to learn how better to manage pain and suffering. Palliative care is an old art, and yet a new frontier as well. Ancient medical duties, too often neglected, can now take advantage of improved techniques.

Equity and a Steady-State Medicine

Constant technological innovation makes it increasingly difficult for governments and other providers to distribute those innovations fairly; doing so is the principal challenge to equity. To give everyone the latest and the best, which more often than not means the most expensive as well, is an obvious problem for the poorer developing countries of the world. But it can be a source of friction in developed countries as well. The rising cost of care for those with AIDS, with new drug combinations (protease inhibitors) available to augment AZT, is a case in point. Some states are unwilling or unable to pay those increased costs, estimated at $6,000 to $10,000 a year. Sometimes greater efficiency in the system can allow it to pay for the new technologies. But there is a limit to that strategy, particularly when efficiency efforts have already been exercised on other, similar occasions.

The need to allocate health care resources fairly is well recognized, but remarkably little attention has been focused on the development of technologies that exacerbate the problem of resource allocation in the first place. Outcome assessment alone is inadequate to deal with that problem. There is often a tacit assumption that health care systems are stable entities, perfectly amenable to theories of justice. But it is precisely because they constantly change as a result of technological innovation (sometimes combined with new health emergencies, such as resurgent TB) that they pose such great problems for equitable allocation. If we had exactly and only the same range of technologies as were available twenty or thirty years ago, there would be no problem in equitably allocating resources. We could readily afford that level of medicine and health care. It is in the nature of the case almost impossible to devise an equitable health care system when its technological costs always threaten to outstrip the resources available to pay for them.

A steady-state medicine will have to find a way to break that cycle to achieve equity. It is not enough, for instance, to argue that an equitable health care system should meet the relatively new demand for care of those who have AIDS. Indeed it should—if that will contribute to population health. As I have argued, that should be the new test. Even more money should be invested in education to avoid AIDS in the first

259

place, for example, marked by the stipulation that unlimited funds will not be available to save those who contract the disease. If new technologies are allowed indiscriminately into health care systems, and used with maximum penetration, they will take money away from other needs, and from other patients. A steady-state medicine will choose equity over state-of-the-art technology when a choice must be made.

A sustainable medicine must be a medicine of limits. An equitable medicine must also be a medicine of limits. Put those two perceptions together and the way is open to understand how a steady-state, sustainable medicine will serve many goods at the same time. It will serve the overall good of societies that cannot allow health care progress to hold their health care systems hostage. It will serve the general needs of patients, who need good medicine, not necessarily the latest and best medicine. It will serve the value of equity because it will help make possible a socially affordable medicine.

Designing a Basic Package of Health Care

One way of bringing together the extended argument I have tried to develop in this book is to ask what, given acceptance of the concept of a sustainable, equitable, steady-state medicine, a basic package of health care should be like. This basic package can be provided in three ways: as part of a government program providing full care to its citizens; as part of a government program designed to supplement health care provided by employers or other private programs; and as part of a private, employer-sponsored program providing a full range of services. In Chapter 7, I provided an argument for some dependence upon the market techniques of financial incentives. Yet however the health care is provided, every citizen should have access to a minimally decent plan, a "package" that is adequate and equitable. That package must, at the same time, be sustainable, economically and psychologically. This means it must simultaneously meet most health needs, not all—the "good enough" principle—and that, when it sets limits, it seeks to balance individual and population needs, with a strong bias toward the latter.

This will not be easy. Despite a great deal of talk over the years, there has never been any real progress made toward defining a plausible and affordable basic package of health care benefits. Though various standards have been proposed—among them "a minimum level of adequate care," the provision of "medically necessary care," and "a decent minimum of care"—none have managed to make themselves fully coherent internally, to promise affordability, or to strike a responsive political chord. When the U.S. Congress stated, for instance, in the 1965 Medicaid legislation that the goal of the program would be to provide "medically necessary" care to the indigent, it did not define that concept; nor, in the years since, has any sustained effort been made within the Medicaid program to define it.[13] The net result is that Medicaid is enormously erratic, with coverage and standards varying from state to state. The idea of what is "medically necessary" has neither been explored much in theory nor coherently used in practice. Whatever the full range of reasons for this omission, one reason is surely the conceptual difficulty of specifying a basic standard of care.

Why has the idea of a basic package or a minimal level of care been so hard to clarify and use? A basic mistake is to assume that such a standard can be developed on purely medical grounds and based on some fixed, universal notion of human need. We could, many once believed, determine some common level of medical need for all people, scientifically specifiable, and work outward from there. It has turned out, however, to be impossible to use "medical need" as a single meaningful criterion for a basic health care package. Needs are too subject to cultural influences and technological progress to remain fixed and stable. The design of a basic package should instead be understood as a work of moral,

261

medical, and economic art, blending scientific knowledge, human needs, and available resources. There is thus a fundamentally political dimension to the idea of a basic package, necessitated by the debatable nature of "needs," and by the necessity to allocate available resources. There must be some role for the public and the professionals together to express their own values about what they believe is a minimally adequate level of care. It is necessary also to have some idea of the proper ends and goals of medicine, and what is to be included in the scope of "health" care. Otherwise there is no clear way to determine whether what people desire in the name of health is what they actually need. I have already indicated that a population orientation will call for evidence about the relative statistical risks people run over a lifetime, and that the notion of "need" should be communal rather than individual.

Why have Americans had so much trouble devising an acceptable package while it seems not to have bothered Europeans very much until recently? The reason, I suspect, is that the European health care systems, all of which provide universal health care in one form or another, began shortly after World War II, in a time of relative poverty.[14] Hence, people did not have excessively high expectations about the range of health care benefits; also, the full impact of technological advances had not yet been felt. Those countries began, therefore, with low expectations and a relatively ineffective medicine. Their notion of what was minimally adequate placed a great deal of emphasis on primary care, public health measures, and disease prevention. That was the least expensive, most efficient way to approach their health problems—and I believe it remains the best way.

By contrast, the United States started its search for a decent minimum, for a basic package, much more recently and from a point of great affluence, well-developed high-technology medicine, and high public expectations of medical benefit. We have also had a strange mixed private market–public entitlement system over the years, one that has become more and more expensive, more and more profitable to those who take part in it, and more and more ambitious in its visions and demands. For Europeans, almost any level of health care was initially acceptable, whereas for Americans practically nothing that can be mentioned is ever quite adequate. Europeans started with relatively low expectations and have been able to build up gradually to higher expectations. The American problem is just the opposite: to find a way to bring high expectations down to a more reasonable level.

In Europe most allocation and rationing decisions have historically been made by politicians and experts working together in private, without much public knowledge, much less participation. This makes life considerably simpler for everybody, and the surprising thing is that the public in those countries has not complained all that much. Over the years, European medical and political authorities, with tacit public support, have been willing to tolerate the limiting of technology, the need to wait in queues for some forms of health care, and the idea that one cannot expect perfection of a universal health care system. That helpful psychological base does not exist in the United States. Moreover, it is doubtful that such a paternalistic, antidemocratic means of decision making can be justified any longer, if it ever could. The latest chapter in the European health care story shows a drift toward American problems: more public participation, more technology, more demand, more complaints (even as health status generally continues to improve).

In thinking about a basic package, it is helpful to glance at some models and approaches that have not worked. One common approach has been simply to specify a list of services that ought to be available under any form of universal health care. Thus the report of the bipartisan 1990 congressional Pepper Commission on Comprehensive Health Care stated that a basic package should include "hospital care, surgical care and other in-patient physician services, physician office visits, diagnostic tests, limited mental health services . . . and preventive services."[15] The only qualification for any of those services was in the word "limited," before "mental health" but before nothing else. Yet the problem with the service-oriented approach is that it specifies no limits on what the services might be, and in that respect more or less opens a blank checkbook. If one simply specifies "hospital care" as one of the services, then of course just about anything that goes on in hospitals, including expensive organ transplants repeated time and again for the same patient, would have to be included. The Pepper Commission's is an inherently open-ended and meaningless standard.

Still another approach is to look at medical benefits, seeking to develop a basic package out of known efficacious treatments. The physician and policy analyst David Hadorn has argued that a basic package should provide only treatments that have proven significantly effective after evaluation by technology assessment.[16] He argues that the best way to define "need" is by the availability of some medical treatment to meet that need. He thus would not define as a need any medical condition for which a treatment does not exist, such as an inoperable brain cancer. By thus limiting the basic package concept to the availability of effective treatment, he makes some great strides toward dealing with one aspect of the problem, namely giving people what will actually do them some good. At the same time, this approach seems terribly narrow, in that some medical needs cannot now be met but could be under a future system, and all the quicker if money is allocated for research on them. The successful outcome of such research eventually expands the scope of the basic package, increasing its costs even as it may also increase its benefits.

Moreover, Hadorn is assuming that we have effective technology assessment, which we really do not at present, and that we can afford to pay for whatever proves to be technologically efficacious. This latter assumption I call the affordability fallacy: because something works it is therefore affordable. Just because the present system includes considerable waste and unnecessary costs, it does not follow that we could therefore afford unlimited expenditures on useful, even cost-effective treatment.

The physician and policy analyst David Eddy has advanced another strategy.[17] His method is to determine what kind of medical care the average person would want and then use that as a standard for determining "essential" care. There would then be developed a "majority choice by average patients," preceded by the effort of a commission to provide good data for people to think about in making their choice.[18] The problem with this approach is that "essential" is defined independently of resources; what the average person would want might well turn out to be unaffordable in the future, and may be so even now. A program of this kind would have to require some educational component to help assure that people had reasonable desires, and of course it would also have to take account of the fact that some desires might still be unreasonable, but would nonetheless have to be factored into the "majority choice." Nonetheless, Eddy's approach underscores both the importance of public participation in designing a package and the inevitable political nature of such a process. As matters now stand, it is increasingly the managers and owners of managed-care organizations that determine the basic package; considerations of competition and cost control reckon heavily in their calculus.

Any discussion of the future of the American health care system will have to take account of public opinion, which will influence the legislative possibilities. The American public is highly confused, divided, and ambivalent about that future, as the collapse of the 1993–1994 health care reform effort made clear. On the one hand, public opinion surveys indicate that most Americans are reasonably satisfied with their own health care, though at the same time they are highly critical of the American health care system in general.[19] Of late, more people have become anxious about the future of their health care, and are particularly concerned about the possibility of losing health care if they change, or lose, a job.

265

The rush to managed care, on the whole supported (according to opinion polls) by the public, is also generating much criticism, which cites the weakening of the doctor-patient relationship, worries about declining quality, and bureaucratic interference with doctors' practice; there is a general dismay at the corporatization of medicine. People remain interested in and generally accepting of national health insurance, but there is little legislative or popular momentum for significant reform. When it is specified that the costs might be high, or that there might be a limitation on the choice of physician, or that people might have to wait for some services, the interest in a universal plan declines considerably. People are willing to see government play a stronger role in controlling the cost of drugs, physician and other health care worker fees, and hospital costs—but they are also deeply suspicious of government management of the overall health care system. Legislators feel that they lack public support on this issue, in great part because the public is not willing to pay much more money for a better or more equitable health care system, but also because people are not certain that their money would be well or efficiently spent even if they did make it available.

Most needed is a different way of providing health care in this country, one that moves away from the enormous fragmentation of the present system toward a more nuanced combination of universality and subsidiarity (local control of small units). One advantage of the present managed-care experiment in the United States is that it has introduced the idea of limits, cost control, central management and efficiency standards, and the need to limit choice as the price of affordability. If the managed care movement could encompass the entire population, it could offer an affordable route to equity. There are no hints of a movement in that direction at present.

Health and the Common Good

Let me try to sketch what might be a possible approach to devising a basic package of health care benefits, and then see whether something like that might be conceivable in this country.

The very first step must be a broad-ranging national discussion of the relationship of health to other societal needs. What should be the overall societal priorities? A great advantage of the budgeting method of the British National Health Service is that health needs must directly compete against other social needs. From the very first, in 1947, the system was designed to make certain that health care did not have a special, privileged position, and that health care expenditures would face off directly with expenditures for housing, transportation, defense, and the like.[20] I believe a system of this kind is necessary in this country as well. Determining the relative priorities among health and other needs requires a basic consideration of the goals and ends of medicine, and the relationship between health and human happiness. These are hardly easy subjects for public discussion, but over a period of years they could be discussed and some rough agreement conceivably reached. Should we have a broader or more limited notion of health? Should health be tightly restricted to physical conditions, or should it move out broadly into general well-being, including many issues of mental health that might otherwise be thought of as nonmedical? These are the kinds of questions that need open public discussion and debate.

If, in an ideal world, health would be compared with other societal goods in the competition for resources, it is important to recognize as well that the design of a health care system must reflect the particular values and culture of the society in which it is developed. In thinking about health in relation to other goods, and in thinking about the comparative allocation of resources *within* health care, some necessary background assumptions must be made. Health care must be culture sensitive, reflecting the values of the people who will pay for the system and use it. However attractive other national systems may be, they cannot be brought wholesale to this country; each grew up in its own native soil. Health care must also be resource relative. It is possible to imagine a health care system that would not be based on the available resources, but to design such a system would be foolish.

Despite the priority I want to give to population health and comparative statistical risks to individuals, a health care system must be alert to variation in individual need. This can be difficult when allocating resources, because for the most part resource allocation is best based on general societal needs; it is exceedingly difficult to tailor national policies to an enormous range of individual variations. Nonetheless, a health care system that was not sensitive to—which is not the same as captured by—those individual variations would neither gain political acceptance nor be likely to pass ethical muster. In trying to put together a basic package of health care, we must recognize that there could be two very different rationales. One rationale is based on individual medical need and the overall welfare of the individual. We could begin by asking what is a necessary minimum of health care for individuals. We could recognize that we ought to share our common fate of pain, illness, and mortality, and that a health care system should express human solidarity in the face of these individual burdens. If we chose to use the individual, and individual need, as the point of departure, we would of course be operating in a way compatible with the values of our culture, and we would also be recognizing that pain and suffering are essentially individual phenomenon.

Yet it is exactly that rationale which is not easily made compatible with equity: too much sensitivity to individual need and variation threatens the common good. We could instead, therefore, look at health in terms of the need to have healthy citizens in order that the institutions and groups of the society might function well. The American public education system, when it was founded in the middle of the nineteenth century, was not designed essentially to help individual children to flourish. It was developed out of a recognition that the economic and social well-being of a country depend upon an educated citizenry. The goal was the common good or the public interest, not the particular good of the individuals to be educated. A similar approach is possible with health care. We can simply ask what level of health a society needs for its economy, schools, families, and so on to function well, and then develop a plan that promotes (at least) that level of health.

I have been drawn to this latter way of thinking because of the history of most European health care systems. The majority of the national health insurance systems on the European continent were not developed out of a rationale of individual rights, but rather for the sake of the common good. European health care is based on public welfare, not on individual rights. In this country, we see such a model in the police and fire departments. In the case of police and fire protection, each of us gets basic protection—but there is no particular provision for individual variation. If I am in a wheelchair, living in a wooden house, I will not get any better service from the fire department than my able-bodied neighbor who lives in a stone house. The same fire department will service all, and if I want additional protection because of my special problems, I must buy it on my own. The same is true of police protection. People accept that model because it is egalitarian, and because it ensures a minimum level of protection for all. We could think of a health care system in the same way. That would place the priority on good public health services and good primary and emergency care. Individuals would have to buy whatever additional care they needed.

Yet as much as I am attracted to a population health model, it is not quite sufficient by itself. We must find a middle ground between an individual-centered and a population-centered standard for provision of health care, but with a new bias in favor of the latter. In seeking a middle way, it is helpful to work with a set of fundamental priorities. I would begin with a nontechnological standard, that of the need to care for individuals. By "care" I mean to focus on the emotional and social needs of the ill, not simply their medical needs. Since medicine is a finite science, and since cure will always finally run out, all of us will at some point in our life need caring.

We need a health care system whose first priority is that no one be abandoned, particularly those whom medicine cannot cure. This, of course, would invert our present priorities, which give cure and the saving of life pride of place. The second priority would be to take measures, well known by now, that promote the public health: immunization, screening, health promotion and disease prevention. The third priority would be to offer primary and emergency care. It is well known from the experience of other countries that a high ratio of primary care physicians to specialists is a good way to keep the public healthy as well as to be sensitive to individual medical needs. That is an important contribution of the managed-care movement, which has adopted that strategy. Everyone will need primary and emergency care at some time during his or her life, and not only does that kind of care often save life, but it provides the necessary basis for determining what is wrong with the patient and what might best be done. Primary care also provides a powerful reassurance to people. They know there will always be someone to deal with their medical problems.

The fourth priority would be advanced technological medicine, of a kind that we find in elaborate forms of surgery, chemotherapy, and the like. The fifth and final health priority would be highly advanced technology, of the kind exemplified by organ transplantation, kidney dialysis, and open-heart surgery. I put advanced technologies and highly advanced technologies last on my list both because they are expensive and because they provide more benefit to individuals than to society as

270

a whole. They are not the main ingredients in keeping up a high level of public health, although they can make some contribution.

In sum, by placing caring first, then moving on to those things designed to help the broadest possible public, and then giving the last priority to advanced forms of technological medicine, I signal an effort to find a good balance between individual and societal emphases.

At the same time, of course, it will be necessary in developing a basic package to be prepared to have some other broad priorities; inevitably, there will be competition for funds. It is reasonable to give priority to the young over the old, to the poor over the rich (particularly in government programs), to those responsible for the care of others over single people, and to those whose race, gender, or ethnic background have placed them at a higher-than-average risk for illness and death. Those best off at present do not need better health care or more medical progress, but the worst off do, to bring them up to a decent standard of care. It is perfectly legitimate to use cost-benefit calculations and other economic tools as long as they are not wholly dominant. They should be a tool, not the kind of technical device used by itself to make a decision.

In sketching some of the ingredients of a basic package, I do not want to neglect a fundamental question. How should we, as individuals, think about our own health care needs—our personal responsibility for health—and what should we ask of our society by way of meeting those needs? Politics will be determined by citizen participation, and citizens will bring their wants and desires to that process. So what ought I to *want* and *desire* as a citizen, as a person? What should we encourage people to think about in their own lives?

I will not try to give a full answer to those questions here, but let me at least suggest some general points. In the first place, the individual needs to think about the place of health in his or her own life. What kind of priority should it have as a personal good? We all understand that there are both hypochondriacs, who give health far too important a place, and other people who are much too careless about their health. There must be a good balance struck here, and it is important for individuals to think about what it should be.[21] They should also think about the place of health in our society. How much emphasis should we place on health in comparison with other needs? Even if health is a necessity for the pursuit of other goods, does that mean it always trumps those other goods? Health is a means to human goods, not an end in itself; a society needs only as much good health as will ensure its civic functioning. A good society does not require perfect health, nor do we as individuals.

Morally speaking, one can see three different demands or claims being made for health care and raising basic questions of equity. There can be a claim upon myself, i.e., the duty I have to take care of myself. There can be a claim upon my family to provide me with health care. There can be a claim upon my society for that which neither my family nor I can provide. One fundamental problem in devising a decent and equitable health care policy is to decide how to adjudicate those different claims. Or, to put it another way, to what extent am I responsible for my own health care, to what extent can I make a claim upon my family to help with my health care, and in what ways and to what extent can I make a claim upon society to help me? How do we want to allocate our responsibilities among us as individuals, as members of families, and as citizens?

In making a claim for myself, I can certainly hope to live a long, healthy, and functional life. Yet it is reasonable as a primary obligation to believe that I ought to take care of my own health, both for my own sake and to avoid being an unnecessary burden on others. I ought not knowingly to engage in unhealthy behaviors, even those that seem to affect only myself. In our health care system, and in every other, it is practically impossible to meet a health care need in ways that will not affect others, either directly or indirectly.

What is my claim upon my family? Families ought to provide love and emotional support in my illness, and be prepared to provide some financial support if that is necessary and possible for them. They are, I believe, next in line to do for me what I cannot do for myself. But my claim upon family members cannot be unlimited. I cannot ask of others, as a duty, that they jeopardize their own health and welfare in my behalf. It is of course hard to draw a line here, the line between charity and duty, but we might at least note that there should be such a line.

There is, finally, the claim upon society. What is a reasonable claim there? What can I ask of my fellow citizens in my illness and disability? Society ought to help me to function as a citizen, to relieve my most egregious suffering as an individual, and to give me reasonable access to the health care facilities that are generally accessible to other citizens. To make an unlimited claim upon my society for health care, however, is unreasonable. I have no right to jeopardize the health of others in pursuit of my own needs. I cannot ask for or expect immortality. I cannot ask that my health needs be placed above other important societal needs. I ought not to be a party to an unsustainable medicine. I ought to be willing to run the risk that my particular illness, or the therapy it requires, will lose out to other medical conditions that are more common.

There is now, and will remain, a basic tension between our individual aspirations for improved health and our human reality as finite beings. Scientific progress guarantees that medicine will continue raising its sights about what it can do for us, and thus stimulating us to want more for ourselves than earlier generations might have wanted for themselves. I can ask to live a reasonably long life in order to make my contribution as a citizen, but I cannot claim that I need any additional life beyond the present average life expectancy of seventy-five to eighty-two in order that we will have a good society. If most of us can live into old age, though not into an ancient old age, we will have lived long enough to guarantee our fellow citi-

273

zens our active participation in our common life. This is only to say that we do not need unlimited medical progress to have a decent and equitable common health. It is also to say that we cannot have an equitable common health if we pursue unlimited progress.

CHAPTER NINE

Sustainable Medicine, Sustainable Hope

Can human beings live without hope? The Roman stoics thought so in ancient times, Buddhists for many centuries now, and some existentialists in more recent days. Yet far more striking in the historical record is the apparent universality and persistence of hope as an enduring human need. It was surely central to the ancient Hippocratic tradition, which required that the physician keep hope alive even if death was clearly on its way. In modern secular hands the need for hope has taken scientific and political forms, often messianic in their aims.

Medicine in particular transferred from the realm of the sacred to that of the secular the longing to redeem and transform the body, otherwise doomed to decay and death. Modern medicine has held out the hope that the biology of the body, and perhaps even of the mind, can be mastered and dominated, that suffering can be relieved and that there is no outer boundary of the possible. The considerable enough progress medicine has so far made toward fulfilling that promise has seemed to encourage the constant stimulation of hope, even to demand it, as if we could not live well without it.

This book has been an argument against unbounded hope. While it served useful purposes earlier, overcoming an excessive fatalism, it is the wrong hope now, skewed and outdated. It will not serve sick people in the next historical era of medicine. We need, instead, to take medicine back to its own roots in the tradition of *hygeia*, which was pushed aside by that scientific medical tradition which has acted as if nature can be pushed aside. But I want to rephrase my original question. I do not doubt that we human beings need hope, in some form or other—though perhaps some of us need it more than others—and I do not doubt that modern medicine has supplied it in ample measure. My more pointed question, pertinent to medicine, is this: can human beings—can we—live without unbounded and limitless hope, of a kind that has no final resting place, which is almost and perhaps necessarily infinite in its longing? That is the form of hope inspired by modern medicine. Could we—can we—should we—settle for something less?

The premise of religious hope has been the need to satisfy a yearning for the infinite, for unity with the transcendent, if such there be. All other hopes and desires are seen as temporary, flawed, mere hints or premonitions of something more, much more. Religion, at least Western religion, can settle for nothing less than unbounded hope to match unbounded longing. The secular hopes of scientific medicine seem to have shared a parallel aspiration. By positing a never-ending quest for improvement, for something always more than whatever it is we now have in our biological makeup, medicine has at times seemed a religion manqué. It has a deep faith in science and an unrestricted hope in the future, and it professes an abiding love for human beings and their welfare.

It would be foolish to suggest that medicine give up its

hope for *something* better in the future. I doubt that would ever be possible as long as illness, pain, suffering, and death are part of human life, as they always will be. But what should count as "better"? That has been the subject of this book. Nor am I proposing that medicine wholly give up its faith in science, though it might be better off a little more skeptical about the possibilities of finding the ultimate causes of human disease, and perhaps a trifle less worshipful in its homage to science (there are other fruitful ways of thinking about human welfare). Least of all would I (or anyone else) want a medicine less than fully enamored of human beings and what can usefully be done to relieve their estate.

No, it is that unbounded and unlimited hope I am after—that hope without end. Hope without end is a religious quest, but not appropriate or sensible for medicine. In its place, I have tried to suggest some alternative possibilities, hopes that have an imaginable and feasible endpoint. But could such finite hopes—either mine or anyone else's—ever satisfy most people? Or, to return to the way I tried to define a sustainable medicine at the beginning of this book: could a steady-state medicine be psychologically sustainable? This is a far more difficult problem than that of developing an economically sustainable medicine. The latter might come about one way or another whatever we do, either through sheer, nasty resource limitation or through its equivalent, an unwillingness of people or societies to pay more for better medicine or better health care even if they might like to have it.

Psychological sustainability is another matter. It is all but ignored save for some oblique hints in public opinion surveys about levels of patient satisfaction with the quality of their health care. That is not quite what I have in mind. The satisfaction I want to specify lies in whether medicine in its present and near-future state meets people's deepest hopes for their mental and physical well-being, whether it satisfies their desire for a life less threatened by or burdened with illness, disability, and death—with the finitude of their bodies. No one, so far as

I know, has ever tried to measure this, but to judge from rhetoric and medical behavior the answer would seem to be no. Whatever medicine has given people so far, they want still more. If cancer has run in their family (as colon cancer runs in my mother's family), they want it eradicated. If heart disease threatens their lives, they want something done about it (and, as the leading cause of death, heart disease threatens almost everyone's; it killed my wife's father). If the prospect of Alzheimer's disease casts a shadow over their old age, they want it eliminated (and who does not, these days, know of someone with that disease?).

It is hardly astonishing, then, that misery can easily be found. Nor should we be surprised that the research agenda of medicine, with considerable public support, is constituted as if unlimited dissatisfaction, unease, and anxiety abound, about which something can and must be done. That part of the human condition influenced by nature and biology—that is, most of the human condition—is not yet satisfactory, far from it. But it is not clear what, if anything, would count as "satisfactory."

There is a puzzle here. How could medicine *ever* be satisfactory if the kind of progress it pursues posits no final resting place, but keeps upping the ante, raising standards for what should count as satisfactory as progress is made from one stage to another? It has not always been that way. Before modern medicine, some peace was made with the finitude of the body—never a perfect peace, but one that allowed people to find some meaning in a life marked by disease and death. Modern medicine, by banishing fatalism and, in effect, declaring the hope of progress to be an essential ingredient in the quest for meaning, changed all that. The earlier search for a meaning to be given to pain and suffering was supplanted by an all-out struggle against them. To look for meaning is already to be fatalistic, an especially grievous sin. The modern point is to eliminate pain and suffering; any amount of them, and any risk of them, is too much.

There is still another puzzle here. To the extent that medicine makes its peace with the market as a political ideology and as a way of paying for the high costs of health care, there can be no satisfactory resting place either. The market, no less than the idea of medical progress, has no endpoint. It exists to serve individual preferences, whatever they might be — it is not for the market, lacking a soul, to judge — and the market offers a way, so goes the claim, of serving those preferences in the most freedom-enhancing way. The market is an impersonal medium of exchange, and that is taken to be its special strength, rewarding competition, blessing efficiency, praising choice.

When the market idea, moreover, is hitched to the romance of technological innovation, then social prosperity more generally is said to be advanced: health care means local jobs, medical technology can profitably be exported, progress pays. But in that context, the notion of psychological sustainability — a steady, slowly innovating or noninnovating state — becomes anathema. It is like asking fish to live in a desert. If people have been tutored to look for progress without end and progress without final goals, they have no less been tutored to think that whatever technology we have now, whether medical or automotive or communicative, is as nothing compared to what we will have, and deserve to have, in the future.

Add now to this mix another demigod of developed societies: liberal individualism. It eschews altogether any belief that we either can or should find something that looks like the human good, some essential human condition to which we should all aspire. Psychological sustainability thereby receives yet another blow. That kind of sustainability would require that we find some conceivable common good and resting place in a medicine that no longer sought infinite progress and the unconstrained transcendence of our limited bodies, those bodies that are a nice token of all our other limitations. A political philosophy that can make no space for substantive public discourse on the good life, or human ends, or the virtues we need to live worthy private lives, can have no space for that kind of medicine either.

A medicine with substantive and limited ends in mind would in fact be a threat, looking within our biology for intrinsic ends and values officially banished from consideration in the larger society. If a thin theory of the good is thought to be the only acceptable political theory, it will not do for so influential a social institution as medicine to subversively reject it. But of course psychological sustainability cannot be nourished, or really be kept alive at all, in that climate, cool and dry, like a Mongolian desert with unlimited horizons.

Then there is nature. If nature is utterly meaningless, offering no guides or directions, hints or suggestions, for the living of a life—if nature represents just so much inchoate stuff to be used as we see fit, utterly adaptable to our purposes—then psychological sustainability loses its last possible toehold. There ceases to be any reason why medicine should not aspire to whatever the public—or those who like profit, or just seek something different—wants it to aspire to. And then, with that achieved, medicine may as well find something more to aspire to, and so on forever, always pushing on. Nothing stands in the way. Nature, once the great and impregnable barrier to human aspiration, is now thought to be wholly malleable, requiring some prudence in its management but not much more.

What is the result of that way of thinking? An infinitely manipulable nature, worked on by an innovation-loving market, which is undergirded by a political philosophy that has disavowed a discovery of human ends, offers not a shred of possibility for psychological sustainability. Even with the nastiest of market pressures, it makes economic sustainability almost impossible as well.

Modest Hopes

These are formidable obstacles to a sustainable medicine. I have tried to offer some alternative forms of hope: a more modest view of progress, a more realistic assessment of the possibilities of technological innovation, a more sober, ecologically tutored understanding of nature. These seem to me worthy and attainable hopes, shed of the grandiose flavor of the expansionary medicine that has marked our era. The policy alternatives I have laid out as an approach to a sustainable medicine—assuming we can change many other values along the way—may seem to have an austere flavor: a public health and population approach that will leave some people floundering (though not utterly sinking) in its wake, even if the overall outcome is egalitarian and the general health is improved, and an emphasis on personal responsibility that will not come easily to many (including me).

My proposed approach is not as austere as it looks. Most of us in the developed countries are already in decent health. Most of our babies no longer die (though one of mine did), most mothers will not die in childbirth either (though a daughter-in-law of mine did), most of us will make it through middle age (though some of my friends did not), and most of us will live well into old age before being brought down (though my father did not get that far). Despite the exceptions, all the odds are in our favor: most babies, most childbearing women, most middle-aged adults make it through a long life. Much of what I have been advocating, save for the diminishing of technological medicine, has come our way already. Not all of us are healthy, but enough of us are to see an endpoint— if, that is, we are looking for an endpoint, as I am.

Patently, the steady-state medicine I espouse runs up against a wide range of other values and proclivities. They have thoroughly infiltrated medicine as an institution and have helped shape the way it thinks about its own ends and goals. To ask that there still be hope, but finite hope, and that those hopes be attached to finite goals that might be achieved and might represent a resting point, seems in one sense not to be asking too much. But in the eyes of many it will seem an extravagantly depressing demand—those in the throes of the endless evil of illness, death, and physical or mental suffering, who are not comforted by the advances so far made, who are more aware of what might yet be done than what has already been achieved. They include the young woman dying of breast cancer, the struggling spouse of an Alzheimer's victim, the young man afflicted by HIV disease; the list is long. There is now a proposal before Congress to double the budget of the National Institutes of Health over the next decade, a remarkable proposal in an era of budget cuts and budget balancing— but understandable enough if one's perception is that of great unmet needs and great possibilities of progress.

I acknowledge that way of looking at things. I have no choice. It is shared by the people I know and respect, and surely pervasive among the general public. I readily concede that the entertainment of finite hopes must include, in its reckoning, not just reduced hope but also the permanent continuation of suffering from our biological frailties. This will necessarily come about if a sustainable medicine is taken seriously, because of the progress forgone, the innovations not pursued, the health budgets not increased, the risks and imperfections left in place, the ragged edge of progress accepted. I believe it is what we would get *anyway*, even if we pursued the present unlimited kind of hope. At least the latter offers us the always sweet tonic of hope itself, admitting no fixed obstacles, and that seems to be what many people, including the visionaries of medical research, need.

I concede, then, that the policy strategy I think will best serve us—combining the impersonality of a public health and population-based approach with a demand for personal responsibility—will for the moment leave some individual health needs unmet, even if it should in the long run reduce such needs. The body goes wrong and people die early even if care is taken of it. Technology and therapeutic medicine, aesculapian in their thrust, will be standing eagerly by to set things right. That thrust must be curbed, even if it goes against the grain to do so. I look to a judicious use of market incentives, especially a requirement to pay something out of our own pockets, to dampen technological enthusiasm—*dampen* it, not extinguish it.

Even so, the ideal of psychological sustainability will be under heavy pressure. And why not, since sick people will want what might make them well—even if they recognize that, since death comes to us all, they will eventually lose. The achievement of a sustainable medicine will mean that they will have to give up, as the first step, the hope that those desires can always be met. In the environmental movement, I note, there is a tension analogous to the psychological sustainability I have tried to describe. The rich nations of the world, with high living standards and long life expectancies, consume a disproportionately large portion of the earth's resources and contribute an excessively large portion of its pollution. Not only will it be necessary to persuade those rich countries to live in an environmentally less profligate fashion, it is also necessary to ask the poor countries to forgo seeking many of the goods of life now enjoyed by the rich countries. That seems to the latter an intolerable demand, unjust on its face, even if the price of achieving equality is an unsustainable environment.

There is no happy way to avoid that tension—though one can see, in the responses to it, the same faith in technological innovation as a magic bullet that is seen in medicine when it is faced with rising costs and burdensome social demands and dilemmas. In any case, just as sick people are not likely to take kindly to a sustainable medicine that might leave them losers, so also the poor countries of the world are not likely to welcome a sustainable-environment movement that asks them to stay behind those who are better off. Neither are those already well off from the exploitation of the environment likely to want to scale back, or those used to state-of-the-art "high-quality" medicine likely to be willing to settle for something less.

Evil and Health

How can all of them, rich and poor, be led to think differently about the medicine of the future? The poor have every reason to want to be as healthy as those who at present are well off. That demand must be acknowledged. Yet it is perfectly possible that, with the strategy I have outlined, they could achieve their goal in far less expensive and socially draining ways than have the affluent they now envy. A strong effort to improve public health and health promotion programs, combined with a rising level of education and economic well-being, could do that job. The poor should not, however, ask that the health status they want be achieved, if necessary, by expanding the reach and intensity of technological medicine. Neither they nor anyone else can afford much more of that. To insist on it in the name of parity would hurt the poor as well as the rich in the long run.

The affluent, the well-off, the already fairly healthy are the real problem. They are never happy, never satisfied with just enough, addicted to progress, never willing to run risks when risks might be reduced. What can be said to them? I have tried to make three general appeals: that *no* society can any longer economically afford to entertain the idea of unlimited progress; that there are better ways to improve health than a heavy dependence upon technological medicine; and that we will all have better health if we think in terms of the welfare of whole communities and populations than if we pursue individual benefits. This is the way to a sustainable medicine. And if we pursue individual benefits, we will not in the long run actually provide them anyway; that is our dilemma.

I want to add one more consideration, bearing on the way the evils of illness and death are thought about. If medicine, particularly on the research side, is to help foster its own sustainability, it must find a way to rid itself of the reigning belief that only eradication of the evil of illness and disease is a worthy goal. This is a mistaken goal. As the resurgence of infectious disease and the stubbornness of chronic disease should make clear, we cannot finally eradicate illness and death. We can only delay them a bit and make their impact less nasty. Medicine will, forever I believe, have to live with that reality, which is given us by nature and will not be eliminated from nature. Hence, when medicine thinks about medical progress, or technological innovation, that permanent reality has to be given a serious place—and not just in palliative-care and hospice programs, where at least some serious movement toward an acceptance of death is taking place.

As important as that movement is, it is not enough; it can still leave in place, utterly untouched, the research imperative to conquer the causes of death and to eliminate the sources of pain and suffering. The restless unhappiness behind that imperative needs some palliative care. If pain, suffering, and illness cannot be conquered or eliminated, as they cannot, then modern medicine must find at its very center a place to permanently coexist with the evils that can be visited upon the body and the mind.

In what might that coexistence consist? Here I can only offer an agenda for further reflection, a direction in which to go:

1. *Rethinking the Problem of Medical Evil.* Are pain and suffering evil, and, if so, what kind of evil? Surely they are evil, at least in the sense that they bring us misery as individuals, often cut us off from others if their intensity is too great, and offer no immediate benefits. I am tempted to exclude here those evils we knowingly bring upon ourselves. But that will not altogether do. For I take it to be one of the glories of medicine that it treats all the sick alike even when they may be morally undeserving; medicine does not care about that. I take it also to be one of the glories of our humane nature that we can, in our better moments, feel empathy even for those who suffer from

their own faults and bad behavior: we are able to see ourselves in them, at least if we have a little imagination.

Now, if we agree that there is evil in the pain and suffering brought on by biological causes, what kind of evil is it? Even if some of the evil is avoidable, much of it is not and never will be. It is simply part of the way things are. In that case, medicine would do well to understand that its task must be to help people live with that evil, not fool themselves into thinking that it can someday be utterly eliminated. Medicine can thus help relieve suffering, and that is a perfectly legitimate response: to lighten suffering's impact. Medicine can also, by shifting its research aims away from the modern struggle against death as its highest priority, move toward improving the quality of life, enhancing life within a finite span. It can see palliative medicine and the care of the dying not just as what is done when all else fails—a permanent second best—but as the very heart of the medical enterprise. We are all likely, after all, to need it, something that can be said about few other medical skills. Medicine's new task will be to give up its triumphalist march toward the eradication of all biological evil, a hopeless venture, and instead call a permanent truce. A truly sustainable medicine will decide that it can never wholly win and, with that thought in mind, will work to find ways to live with, even as it struggles with, evil. If we believe that death should be clinically understood as a part of life—which we all say these days—then we must also accept illness, the cause of death, as a part of life. They go together, but we have pretended they can be separated.

2. *Meaning and the Human Good.* In an earlier chapter, I argued that a sustainable medicine will have a tough time of it in societies that have banished, or remain fearful of, a public reflection upon the human good. A medicine that cannot anchor itself in any consensus about the nature of human needs, or the ends of human life, cannot set any coherent goals for itself. Its inner life will be as open to the highest bidder as the

cultural life of the societies in which it is embedded. This is all
the more unfortunate in the case of a medicine struggling with
the evil of disease and death, two aspects of human life that
call out for understanding and meaning. A medicine which
says, in effect, that death and disease have no meaning and
must simply be eliminated—in a society that says it can make
no sense of them either and must abandon them to our hidden, private lives—is a medicine that offers no common rationale for sustainability. Everything is left to political process on
the one hand, divorced from moral substance and depth, and
to individual choice and direction on the other, sundered from
any connection with a recognizable common good.

Medicine must find a way out of this impasse. It must re-
connect itself to the search for meaning, to the devising of social and cultural rituals for coping with sickness and death,
and to the discovery of its place within the hierarchy of institutions designed to help people live better lives. Medicine now
gives science the privileged place in its methodology and its attempt to understand the body and the mind. Science *should*
always have a high place. But its privileged rank has driven to
the margins the insights of religion, the humanities, folk and
traditional cultures, and those psychological and social sciences that look for ways to overcome the duality of mind and
body, of individual and culture, of illness and societal values.
There is a great stirring these days in all these domains, and
the insights they offer should be taken seriously, though never
uncritically. Those developments offer the possibility that people will learn how better to live with illness, how better to live
healthy lives, how better to manage the fact of limits and finitude. That could be a major contribution to the psychological
sustainability of an economically steady-state medicine.

3. *Toward Medicine's Third Era.* Early in this book, I set forth
the possibility of a new, third era of medicine, an era marked
by a change in some of medicine's modern reigning values
and, especially, by sustainability as a new value. I have already

granted that an untrammeled market could force a sustainable medicine—no one would get what they could not or would not pay for—but I believe that a sustainability so achieved would have tragic individual and social consequences. It is bad enough to deal with the woes of the body, much less to deal with them while burdened with economic anxiety, which is just what happens when the market is given too much play.

A new, third era of medicine would require a far better merging than at present of the search for population and individual health. But we have yet to find a good way to understand the relationship between individual medical good and population medical good. The latter has seemed distant and impersonal, nice enough, but only up to a point. For a population perspective to make a serious difference, we must develop much greater public and professional understanding of the way living in common, sharing a public environmental, economic, and social life, affects individual health. Concern with environmental hazards touches on this, as does the fresh focus on the role of stress in our work and family life.

This is only to say that a third-era medicine, marked by sustainability, will have to be at once more limited in its aspirations for progress, more tolerant of the need to accept some evil, and more open and imaginative, farther-ranging in its ways of making sense of the human medical condition. A sustainable medicine is necessary not simply because we cannot afford any other but also because it could help displace the goal-less, progress-driven, never-happy medicine that came out of medicine's embrace of modernism. A sustainable medicine will force a reconsideration of the body and mind, of the social meaning of medicine and health care, and of the relationship of medicine to the cultures of which it is a part. If an economically sustainable medicine is to be psychologically sustainable as well, that is the only possible direction for it.

The long-standing presumption of modern medicine has been that more and better medicine equals more and better health. That is not true, even if medicine can make important contributions to individual health. Yet there is another presumption that has not received comparable scrutiny: that the more health people have, the happier they will be. This does not seem to be true either, though no doubt medicine can help happiness along at some points. It should more generally be clear that happiness requires a good society, a community of decent people, jobs, education, housing, and peace. Health is only one ingredient of individual and social happiness. Medicine, which has seen itself as having a special role in producing happiness, now needs to take the broader view. It has already brought us a long way, and that is eminently creditable. Now it needs to reconceive its role, understanding that our chance of happiness is not necessarily enhanced by more medical advances, but rather by whether those advances serve all the other human needs and aspirations. That seems to me the important test.

Notes

PREFACE

1. Robert Blendon, Kaiser Harvard Program, Press Release, June 30, 1996.
2. Paul B. Ginsburg and Jeremy Pickreign, "Tracking Health Care Costs: An Update," *Health Affairs*, Vol. 16 (July-August 1997), pp.151–155; see also "Low-Cost Trends Continued in 1996," *Issue Briefs* (June 1997), pp. 1–4, which notes the likelihood of a 4–5 percent increase in 1998, over against a general 3 percent annual inflation rate; Foster Higgins, "Health Costs May Be Heading Up Again," *Business and Health Magazine* (1997), p. 8.
3. The World Bank, *Investing in Health: World Development Report 1993* (New York: Oxford University Press, 1993).
4. World Health Organization, *Renewing the Health-for-all Strategy* (Geneva, Switzerland: World Health Organization, 1995).
5. The Hastings Center, "The Goals of Medicine: Setting New Priorities," *Hastings Center Report*, Vol. 26, Supplement (November–December 1996), pp. 1–32.
6. René Dubos, *Mirage of Health: Utopias, Progress, and Biological Change* (New York: Harper & Row, 1959).
7. Ivan Illich, *Medical Nemesis: The Expropriation of Health* (New York: Pantheon, 1976).
8. Ibid.; John Powles, "On the Limitations of Modern Medicine," *Science, Medicine & Man*, Vol. 1 (1973), pp. 1–30; Rick J. Carlson, *The End of Medicine* (New York: John Wiley & Sons, 1975); Thomas

291

McKeown, *The Role of Medicine: Dream, Mirage, or Nemesis*
(Princeton, N.J.: Princeton University Press, 1979).

9. Carlson, op. cit., p. 1.

10. Much of the ensuing discussion, together with an analysis of
other efforts to change the models of medicine, is summarized and developed in Kerr L. White, *The Task of Medicine: Dialogue at Wickenburg*
(Menlo Park, Calif.: The Henry J. Kaiser Family Foundation, 1988). The
writings of Dr. White and of George L. Engel are particularly important;
see, for example, Engel's essay "How Much Longer Must Medicine's
Science Be Bound by a Seventeenth Century World View?" in the Kerr
volume, as well as the section "Patient and Population Perspectives" in
the introductory essay. The "tradition" I have identified has now also been
vigorously revived (though it was never quite dead) by Robert G. Evans,
Morris L. Barer, and Theodore R. Marmor, eds., *Why Are Some People
Healthy and Others Not? The Determinants of Health of Populations*
(New York: Aldine de Gruyter, 1994).

ONE: CREATING A SUSTAINABLE MEDICINE

1. World Health Organization, *The World Health Report 1996:
Fighting Disease, Fostering Development* (Geneva, Switzerland: World
Health Organization, 1966), p. v.

2. Joseph Fletcher, *Morals and Medicine* (Princeton, N.J.:
Princeton University Press, 1954), p. 170.

3. René Descartes, "Discourse on the Method of Rightly
Conducting the Reason and Seeking for Truth in the Sciences," in *The
Philosophical Works of Descartes*, trans. Elizabeth S. Haldane and G. R.
T. Ross (Cambridge, England: Cambridge University Press, 1981), p.
120.

4. Harold Varmus, "Shattuck Lecture—Biomedical Research
Enters the Steady State," *The New England Journal of Medicine*, Vol.
333 (September 21, 1995), pp. 811–15.

5. Gail R. Wilensky, "The Score on Medicare Reform—Minus the
Hype and Hyperbole," *The New England Journal of Medicine*, Vol. 333
(December 28, 1995), p. 1774.

6. Rashi Fein, "Assessing the Proposed Medicare Reforms," *The
New England Journal of Medicine*, Vol. 333 (December 28, 1995), p.
1778.

7. George J. Annas, "Reframing the Debate on Health Care
Reform by Replacing Our Metaphors," *The New England Journal of
Medicine*, Vol. 332 (March 16, 1995), pp. 744–47.

8. There is an environmental journal called *Ecosystem Health*; see
also Peter Berman, "Health Sector Reform: Making Health
Development Sustainable," *Health Policy*, Vol. 32 (1995), pp. 13–28,

which interestingly discusses the role of health care in development strategies.

9. Christopher J. L. Murray and Alan D. Lopez have used a life expectancy of 82.5 for females and 80.0 for males as models in measuring the global burden of disease, in *The Global Burden of Disease* (Cambridge, Mass.: Harvard University Press, 1996), pp. 16–18.

10. John Knowles, "Introduction," *Daedalus*, Vol. 106 (Winter 1977), pp. 1–7.

11. The best book on this general phenomenon is still Arthur J. Barsky, *Worried Sick: Our Troubled Quest for Wellness* (Boston: Little, Brown, 1988).

12. David Mechanic, "Emerging Trends in the Application of the Social Sciences to Health and Medicine," *Social Science and Medicine*, Vol. 40 (1955), p. 1492.

13. Lewis Thomas, *The Lives of a Cell* (New York: Bantam Books, 1974), pp. 37–39.

14. René Dubos, *Mirage of Health: Utopias, Progress, and Biological Change* (New York: Harper & Row, 1959).

Two: Arguing with Success: Progress and the Medical Dream

1. Al Gore, "The Metaphor of Distributed Intelligence," *Science*, Vol. 272 (April 12, 1996), p. 177.

2. Quoted in James Thomas Flexner, *Washington: The Indispensable Man* (New York: Little, Brown, 1974), p. 260.

3. Daniel Sarewitz, *Frontiers of Illusion: Science, Technology, and the Politics of Progress* (Philadelphia: Temple University Press, 1996), p. 19.

4. Cited in Richard Wolin, "Liberation as a Vocation," *The New Republic* (September 2, 1996), p. 34.

5. René Descartes, "Discourse on the Method of Rightly Conducting the Reason and Seeking for Truth in the Sciences," in *The Philosophical Works of Descartes*, trans. Elizabeth S. Haldane and G. R. T. Ross (Cambridge, England: Cambridge University Press, 1981), p. 120.

6. G. Michael Fossel, *Reversing Human Aging* (New York: Morrow, 1996), p. 1.

7. Bernadine Healy, "Shattuck Lecture: NIH and the Bodies Politic," *The New England Journal of Medicine*, Vol. 330 (May 26, 1994), p. 1498.

8. Gerald Holton, *Science and Anti-Science* (Cambridge, Mass.: Harvard University Press, 1993), p. 6. The medical examples of the concepts' use are mine, not Holton's.

9. J. B. Bury, *The Idea of Progress: An Inquiry into Its Origin and Growth* (New York: Dover Publications, 1932), p. 7.

10. Thomas Sowell, *A Conflict of Visions* (New York: William Morrow, 1987), pp. 18ff.

11. Cited in Christopher Lasch, *The True and Only Heaven: Progress and Its Critics* (New York: W. W. Norton, 1991), p. 43.

12. Bury, op. cit., p. 351.

13. Robert Nisbet, *History of the Idea of Progress* (New York: Transaction Books, 1983), p. 4.

14. Ibid., p. 5.

15. Ibid.

16. Ibid., p. 8.

17. Gunther S. Stent, *Paradoxes of Progress* (San Francisco: W. H. Freeman, 1978), p. 3.

18. Ivan Klíma, *The Spirit of Prague*, trans. Paul Wileon (London: Granta Books, 1994), p. 153. Václav Havel has made a similar point in Jan Vladislav, ed., *Václav Havel: On Living with the Truth* (London: Faber & Faber, 1987), pp. 138–39, although his critique more directly emphasizes the impersonality and potentially dehumanizing features of the quest for objectivity and universality in science.

19. Lasch, op. cit., p. 13.

20. Ibid., p. 530.

21. Ibid.

22. Ibid., p. 18.

23. I have developed this point in *What Kind of Life: The Limits of Medical Progress* (New York: Simon & Schuster, 1990), pp. 41–57.

24. The World Bank, *World Development Report 1993: Investing in Health* (New York: Oxford University Press, 1993), p. 23. That gain is proportionately comparable to the gains in the developed countries.

25. K. C. Manton and Burton Singer, "What's the Fuss About Compression of Mortality?" *Change*, Vol. 7 (1994), pp. 21–30.

26. S. Jay Olshansky, Bruce A. Carnes, and Christine K. Cassel, "The Aging of the Human Species," *Scientific American*, Vol. 268 (April 1993), pp. 46–52; see also, by the same authors, "In Search of Methuselah," *Science*, Vol. 250 (November 2, 1990), pp. 634–40; and Bruce A. Carnes and S. Jay Olshansky, "Evolutionary Perspectives on Human Senescence," *Population and Development Review*, Vol. 19 (December 1993), pp. 793–806.

27. R. H. M. Lohman, K. Sankaranarayanan, J. Ashby, "Choosing the Limits to Life," *Nature*, Vol. 357 (May 21, 1992), pp. 185–86. The authors argue that "as populations . . . approach the maximum average lifespan, health initiatives will result only in a shift in the relative importance of individual causes of death. Thus attempts to extend the average lifespan under such conditions will have only a marginal effect (or none at all) on the average well-being of the population" (p. 185).

28. "Forward to Methuselah," *The Economist* (January 7, 1995), pp.

65–68. As is typical of this genre, the article becomes increasingly less confident as it progresses, piling qualification upon qualification.

29. M. C. Allen, P. K. Donohue, and A. E. Dusman, "The Limit of Viability: Neonatal Outcome of Infants Born at 22 to 25 Weeks' Gestation," *The New England Journal of Medicine*, Vol. 329 (November 25, 1993), pp. 1597–1601.

30. Robert W. Pinner et al., "Trends in Infectious Diseases Mortality in the United States," *Journal of the American Medical Association*, Vol. 275 (January 17, 1996), pp. 189–93.

31. Frank Ryan, *The Forgotten Plague: How the Battle Against Tuberculosis Was Won—and Lost* (Boston: Little, Brown, 1992); Robert F. Breiman et al., "Emergence of Drug-Resistant Pneumococcal Infections in the United States," *Journal of the American Medical Association*, Vol. 271 (June 15, 1994), pp. 1831–35.

32. Laurie Garrett, *The Coming Plague: Newly Emerging Diseases in a World Out of Balance* (New York: Farrar, Straus and Giroux, 1995), p. 451. See also Richard Preston, *The Hot Zone* (New York: Random House, 1995).

33. Institute of Medicine, *Emerging Infections: Microbial Threats to Health in the United States* (Washington, D.C.: National Academy Press, 1992). See also *Report of the NSTC Committee on International Science, Engineering, and Technology (CISET) Working Group on Emerging and Re-emerging Infectious Disease* (Washington, D.C.: National Science and Technology Council, n.d.).

34. Paul W. Ewald, *Evolution of Infectious Disease* (New York: Oxford University Press, 1994), p. 213.

35. Marc Lappé, *Evolutionary Medicine: Rethinking the Origins of Disease* (San Francisco: Sierra Club Books, 1994), p. 211.

36. Dean T. Jamison et al., *Disease Control Priorities in Developing Countries* (Washington, D.C.: The World Bank, 1993), pp. 3–4.

37. Paul G. McGovern et al., "Recent Trends in Acute Coronary Heart Disease," *Journal of the American Medical Association*, Vol. 334 (April 4, 1996), pp. 884–89; American Heart Association, *Heart and Stroke Facts: 1994 Statistical Supplement* (Dallas: American Heart Association, 1994); National Heart, Lung, and Blood Institute, "Data Fact Sheet: Morbidity from Coronary Heart Disease in the United States" (Washington, D.C.: National Institutes of Health, May 1992); Maria G. M. Hunink et al. "The Recent Decline in Mortality from Coronary Heart Disease, 1980–1990," *Journal of the American Medical Association*, Vol. 277 (February 19, 1997), pp. 535–42.

38. John C. Bailor and Heather L. Gornik, "Cancer Undefeated," *The New England Journal of Medicine*, Vol. 336 (May 29, 1997), pp. 1569–74; Michael B. Sporn, "The War on Cancer," *The Lancet*, Vol. 347 (May 18, 1996), pp. 1377–81; American Cancer Society, *Cancer*

Facts & Figures—1994 (Atlanta: American Cancer Society, 1994); Barry A. Miller et al., eds., *SEER Cancer Statistics Review, 1973–1990* (Bethesda, Md.: National Institutes of Health Publication Number 93-2789, 1992); Curtis J. Mettlin, "New Evidence of Progress in the National Cancer Program," *Cancer*, Vol. 78 (November 15, 1996), pp. 6–7.

39. See K. G. Manton, C. H. Patrick, and E. Stallard, "Population Impact of Mortality Reduction: The Effects of Elimination of Major Causes of Death on the 'Saved' Population," *International Journal of Epidemiology*, Vol. 9 (1980), pp. 111–20; Kenneth G. Manton, J. Michael Wrigley, Harvey J. Cohen, and Max A. Woodbury, "Cancer Mortality, Aging, and Patterns of Comorbidity in the United States: 1968–1986," *Journal of Gerontology: Social Sciences*, Vol. 46 (1991), pp. S225–34; Lester R. Curtin and Robert Armstrong, "United States Life Tables Eliminating Certain Causes of Death, 1979–81," Vol. 1 (Washington, D.C.: U.S. Department of Health and Human Services, DHHS Publication No. [PHS] 88-1150-2).

40. S. Jay Olshansky and Bruce A. Carnes, "Demographic Perspectives on Human Senescence," *Population and Development Review*, Vol. 20 (March 1994), p. 76.

41. Antoine-Nicolas de Condorcet, *Sketch for a Historical Picture of the Progress of the Human Mind*, trans. June Berraclough (New York: Library of Ideas, 1955), p. 200.

42. James A. Fries, "The Compression of Morbidity: Near or Far?" *The Milbank Quarterly*, Vol. 67 (1989), pp. 208–232. In this article, Fries appears to have backed down a little from his earlier predictions that a compression of morbidity was likely. Instead, he has shifted the emphasis to the value of *attempting* to reduce morbidity as a sensible and feasible goal of health care. See also James A. Fries, "Aging, Illness, and Health Policy: Implications of the Compression of Morbidity," *Perspectives in Biology and Medicine*, Vol. 31 (Spring 1988), pp. 407–428.

43. Lois M. Verbrugge, "Survival Curves, Prevalence Rates, and Dark Matters Therein," *Journal of Aging and Health*, Vol. 3 (1991), pp. 217–36; Lois M. Verbrugge, "Recent, Present, and Future Health of American Adults," *Annual Review of Public Health*, Vol. 10 (1989), pp. 333–61; S. Jay Olshansky, "Trading Off Longer Life for Worsening Health: The Expansion of Morbidity Hypothesis," *Journal of Aging and Health*, Vol. 3 (May 1991), pp. 194–216. Dorothy Rice, the distinguished statistician, has said of patients with cardiovascular disease that the evidence indicates an increase, not a decrease, in morbidity and increased utilization of both inpatient and outpatient services (Dorothy Rice, personal communication, 1995).

44. Kenneth G. Manton, Larry S. Corder, and Eric Stollard, "Estimates of Change in Chronic Disability and Institutional Incidence

and Prevalence Rates in the U.S. Elderly Population from the 1982, 1984, and 1989 National Long Term Care Survey," *Journal of Gerontology: Social Sciences,* Vol. 48 (1993), pp. S153–66; Kenneth G. Manton, Larry Corder, and Eric Stollard, "Changes in the Use of Personal Assistance and Special Equipment from 1982–1989: Results from the 1982 and 1989 NLTCS," *The Gerontologist,* Vol. 33 (1993), pp. 168–76; Lester Breslow and Norman Breslow, "Health Practices and Disability: Some Evidence from Alameda County," *Preventive Medicine,* Vol. 22 (1993), pp. 86–95. A skeptical analysis of the belief that declines in mortality among the elderly lead to increased frailty and worsening health has been written by Timothy Weidmann, John Bound, and Michael Schoenbaum, "The Illusion of Failure: Trends in the Self-Reported Health of the U.S. Elderly," *The Milbank Quarterly,* Vol. 73 (1995), pp. 253–87.

45. Jeff C. Goldsmith, "The Reshaping of Healthcare," *Healthcare Forum Journal* (May–June 1992), Part I. Cited in "Revolutions and Evolutions in Health Care," *Insight,* December 1994, p. 1.

46. Robert Pollack, *Signs of Life: The Language and Meanings of DNA* (Boston: Houghton Mifflin, 1994), p. 179.

47. Ibid., p. 181.

48. Jeanette M. Smith, "The 'Pennies Drop': Genetic Discoveries of Medical Significance," *Journal of the American Medical Association,* Vol. 270 (November 17, 1993), p. 2370.

49. Ronald Munson and Lawrence H. Davis, "Germ-Line Gene Therapy and the Medical Imperative," *Kennedy Institute of Ethics Journal,* Vol. 2 (June 1992), p. 158; see also Eliot Marshal, "Less Hype, More Biology, Needed for Gene Therapy," *Science,* Vol. 270 (September 15, 1995), p. 1751.

50. P. A. Baird, "The Role of Genetics in Population Health," in *Why Are Some People Healthy and Others Not?* Robert G. Evans, Morris L. Bauer, and Theodore R. Marmor, eds. (New York: Aldine DeGruyter, 1994), p. 159; see also Edward S. Golub, *The Limits of Medicine* (New York: Times Books, 1994), Chapter 10, pp. 205ff; and Philip Kitcher, *The Lives to Come: The Genetic Revolution and Human Possibilities* (New York: Simon & Schuster, 1996).

51. Cited in Gabriel Gyamati, "The Future of Medicine: An Analytical Framework," in *The Goals of Medicine,* Mark J. Hanson and Daniel Callahan, eds. (Washington, D.C.: Georgetown University Press, 1998).

52. George J. Schieber, Jean-Pierre Pouiller, and Leslie M. Greenwald, "Health System Performance in OECD Countries, 1980–1992," *Health Affairs,* Vol. 13 (Fall 1994), pp. 100–111; see also Organization for Economic Cooperation and Development, *New Directions in Health Policy* (Paris: OECD, 1995), pp. 9–10. In the

United States, there was a short-term slowing of the increase in health care costs—with the impact of HMOs believed to be a major contributor to that development—but an upward shift has happened once again. See Paul Ginsburg and Jeremy Pickreign, "Tracking Health Care Costs," *Health Affairs*, Vol. 15 (Fall 1996), pp. 140–49; and Organization for Economic Cooperation and Development, *The Reform of Health Care Systems: A Review of Seventeen OECD Countries* (Paris: OECD, 1994), p. 37.

53. William B. Schwartz, "The Inevitable Failure of Current Cost-Containment Strategies," *Journal of the American Medical Association*, Vol. 257 (January 9, 1987), pp. 220–24. Though written a decade ago, Schwartz's analysis still seems on target. The prescience of Schwartz's analysis is made clear by reports of an upward swing in HMO costs by the end of 1997.

54. John-Arne Skolbekken, "The Risk Epidemic in Medical Journals," *Social Science and Medicine*, Vol. 40 (1995), pp. 291–305. The "risk epidemic" is no less strong in the popular media.

55. Arthur J. Barsky, *Worried Sick: Our Troubled Quest for Wellness* (Boston: Little, Brown, 1988); see also Arthur J. Barsky and Jonathan F. Borus, "Somatization and Medicalization in the Era of Managed Care," *Journal of the American Medical Association*, Vol. 274 (December 27, 1995), pp. 1831–34.

56. Clifton K. Meador, "The Last Well Person," *The New England Journal of Medicine*, Vol. 330 (February 10, 1994), pp. 440–41.

57. David Freeman Hawke, *Benjamin Rush: Revolutionary Gadfly* (Indianapolis: Bobs-Merrill, 1971), p. 99.

58. Daniel Callahan, "The WHO Definition of Health," *Hastings Center Studies*, Vol. 1 (1973), pp. 77–87.

59. Daniel Sarewitz, *Frontiers of Illusion: Science, Technology, and the Politics of Progress* (Philadelphia: Temple University Press, 1996), p. 194.

60. I developed the image of the "ragged edge" of progress at greater length in *What Kind of Life: The Limits of Medical Progress* (New York: Simon & Schuster, 1990), pp. 63ff.

61. Sarewitz, op. cit., p. 167.

THREE: SUSTAINABLE TECHNOLOGY: A MEDICAL OXYMORON?

1. From *News in Brief* (March 20, 1996), p. a. The theme of the close link between American prosperity and technological innovation, for both domestic and export reasons, is common in the literature urging greater investment in technology research and development, now including medical technology.

2. Marc W. Kischner, Elizabeth Marincola, and Elizabeth Olmsted Teisberg, "The Role of Biomedical Research in Health Care Reform," *Science*, Vol. 266 (October 7, 1994), p. 49.

3. "Revolutions and Evolutions in Health Care: The Promise of Emerging Medical Technologies," *Insight*, December 1994, pp. 1–6.

4. Harold E. Varmus, "Science for the Public Good," *Harvard Magazine*, July–August 1996, p. 62.

5. *The Wall Street Journal*, February 16, 1994, p. A18.

6. A special section of *The Economist* developed at great length all of these benefits. While it was conceded that these developments would raise economic and ethical problems, ready confidence was expressed that case-by-case the combination of a healthier, more productive economy and careful regulatory constraints could well cope with them. *The Economist*, March 19, 1994, Survey, pp. 1–18.

7. William B. Schwartz, "In the Pipeline: A Wave of Valuable Technology," *Health Affairs*, Vol. 13 (Summer 1994), pp. 70–79.

8. "Revolutions and Evolutions in Health Care: The Promise of Emerging Medical Technologies," *Insight*, December 1994, p. 3.

9. Eric J. Cassell, "The Sorcerer's Broom," *Hastings Center Report*, Vol. 23 (November–December 1993), p. 33; see also David J. Rothman, *Beginnings Count: The Technological Imperative in American Health Care* (New York: Oxford University Press, 1997).

10. Ibid., p. 35.

11. Ibid., p. 36.

12. John Powles, "On the Limitations of Modern Medicine," *Science, Medicine & Man*, Vol. 1 (1973), p. 21.

13. Cited by Andrew Hacker, "The Medicine in Our Future," *The New York Review of Books*, June 12, 1997, p. 28. This aspect of technological innovation is altogether ignored by Jeff Goldsmith in a response to the article by William B. Schwartz cited in note 7 above. Schwartz notes the economic hazards of those developments: "In the short term, cost is the paramount issue; in the long term, the successes of biomedical research are likely to produce even more serious problems" (p. 79). In response, Goldsmith argues that "Medical technologies are not inherently cost-increasing," but he presents little evidence to support his claim. "The Impact of New Technology of Health Costs," *Health Affairs*, Vol. 13 (Summer 1994), p. 81.

14. See, for instance, Richard A. Rettig, "The Social Contract and the Treatment of Permanent Kidney Failure," *Journal of the American Medical Association*, Vol. 275 (April 10, 1996), pp. 1123–26.

15. Dale A. Rublee, "Medical Technology in Canada, Germany, and the United States: An Update," *Health Affairs*, Vol. 13 (Fall 1994), pp. 113–17.

16. Burton A. Weisbrod, "Technologies, Incentives, and Health

Care Costs: What Is Our Future?" in *Medical and Biological Engineering in the Future of Health Care*, J. D. Andrade, ed. (Salt Lake City: University of Utah Press, 1994), pp. 76–77.

17. J. M. Eisenberg et al., "Substituting Diagnostic Services: New Tests Only Partially Replace Older Ones," *Journal of the American Medical Association*, Vol. 262 (1989), pp. 1196–1200.

18. Daniel Callahan, *What Kind of Life: The Limits of Medical Progress* (New York: Simon & Schuster, 1990), pp. 101–102.

19. For still another perspective on the dynamics of medical innovation, see A. Mark Fendrick et al., "Understanding the Behavioral Response to Medical Innovation," *The American Journal of Managed Care*, Vol. 2 (July–August 1996), pp. 793–99.

20. Joel E. Miller and Eric F. Bernstein, *Medical Practice Assessment Report: Underevaluated Health Care Technology* (Washington, D.C.: Health Insurance Association of America, March 1989), pp. 14–16.

21. For a general analysis of technology assessment in medicine, see Alan M. Garber, "Can Technology Assessment Control Health Spending?" *Health Affairs*, Vol. 13 (Summer 1994), pp. 115–26.

22. For a comprehensive examination of many of the problems of cost-effectiveness analysis, a crucial part of technology assessment, see David M. Eddy. "Cost Effectiveness Analysis: Is It Up to the Task?" *Journal of the American Medical Association*, Vol. 267 (June 24, 1992), pp. 3342–48.

23. See Donald M. Steinwachs, Albert W. Wu, and Elizabeth A. Skinner, "How Will Outcomes Management Work?" *Health Affairs*, Vol. 13 (Fall 1994), pp. 153–62.

24. See Einer Elhauge, "The Limited Potential of Technology Assessment," *Virginia Law Review*, Vol. 82 (1996), pp. 1525–95. For a skeptical account of the use of clinical guidelines, see Roger D. Feldman, John A. Nyman, and Janet Shapiro, "How Will We Use Clinical Guidelines?" *Journal of Health Politics, Policy and Law*, Vol. 19 (Spring 1994), pp. 7–25; and Sandra J. Tanenbaum, "Knowing and Acting in Medical Practice," *Journal of Health Politics, Policy and Law*, Vol. 19 (Spring 1994), pp. 27–44. David M. Frankford has written more generally, and even more critically, about the effort to bring greater scientific rigor to health care, of which technology and economic assessments are a key part: David M. Frankford, "Scientism and Economism in the Regulation of Health Care," *Journal of Health Politics, Policy and Law*, Vol. 19 (Winter 1994), pp. 773–99.

25. Many of these complications are analyzed in Milton C. Weinstein et al., "Recommendations of the Panel on Cost-effectiveness in Health and Medicine," *Journal of the American Medical Association*, Vol. 276 (October 16, 1996), pp. 1253–58; see also Marthe R. Gold et

al., *Cost-effectiveness in Health and Medicine* (New York: Oxford University Press, 1996).

26. See Peter J. Neumann and Magnus Johannesson, "From Principle to Public Policy: Using Cost-effectiveness Analysis," *Health Affairs*, Vol. 13 (Summer 1994), pp. 206–214. For a general defense of the use of cost-benefit analysis, see Kenneth J. Arrow et al., "Is There a Role for Benefit-Cost Analysis in Environmental, Health, and Safety Regulation?" *Science*, Vol. 272 (April 12, 1996), pp. 221–22; and Robert H. Hahn, *Risks, Costs, and Lives Saved: Getting Better Results from Regulation* (New York: Oxford University Press, 1996).

27. William B. Schwartz, "The Inevitable Failure of Current Cost Containment Strategies," *The New England Journal of Medicine*, Vol. 314 (February 13, 1986), pp. 220–24.

28. See Philip Boyle and Daniel Callahan, "Physicians' Use of Outcome Data," in *Getting Doctors to Listen*, Philip Boyle, ed. (Washington, D.C.: Georgetown University Press, 1997).

29. David M. Frankford, "Managing Clinicians' Work Through the Use of Financial Incentives," *Wake Forest Law Review*, Vol. 29 (1994), pp. 71–105.

30. Christopher Lasch, *The True and Only Heaven: Progress and Its Critics* (New York: W. W. Norton, 1991), p. 48.

31. Renée C. Fox, "Experiment Perilous: Forty-five Years as a Participant Observer of Patient-Oriented Clinical Research," *Perspectives in Biology and Medicine*, Vol. 39 (1996), p. 222.

32. John P. Bunker, Howard S. Frazier, and Frederick Mosteller, "Improving Health: Measuring Effects of Medical Care," *The Milbank Quarterly*, Vol. 72 (1994), pp. 225–58. A more pessimistic account is presented in John B. McKinlay, Sonja J. McKinlay, and Robert Beaglehole, "A Review of the Evidence Concerning the Impact of Medical Measures on Recent Mortality and Morbidity in the United States," *International Journal of Health Services*, Vol. 19 (1989), pp. 181–208; see also Paul G. McGovern et al., "Recent Trends in Acute Coronary Hearth Disease," *The New England Journal of Medicine*, Vol. 334 (April 4, 1996), pp. 884–90.

33. John Powles, "On the Limitations of Modern Medicine," *Science, Medicine & Man*, Vol. 1 (1973), p. 23.

34. Schwartz, op. cit., p. 223.

35. T. R. Marmor, M. L. Barer, and R. G. Evans, "The Determinants of a Population's Health: What Can Be Done to Improve a Democratic Nation's Health Status?" in *Why Are Some People Healthy and Others Not? The Determinants of Health of Populations*, Robert G. Evans, Morris L. Barer, Theodore R. Marmor, eds. (New York: Aldine de Gruyter, 1994), p. 221.

36. This is the general argument of the Evans, Barer, and Marmor

book cited in note 35. John Powles's article "On the Limitations of Modern Medicine" (note 33) remains a succinct and persuasive summation of the modern evidence.

37. Marmor et al., op. cit., p. 221; and Kevin M. White and Samuel H. Preston, "How Many Americans Are Alive Because of Twentieth-Century Improvements in Mortality?" *Population and Development Review*, Vol. 22 (September 1996), p. 422.

38. Robert G. Evans and G. L. Stoddard, "Producing Health, Consuming Health Care," in Evans, Barer, and Marmor, op. cit., p. 39.

39. Ibid., p. 40.

40. This general issue is skillfully discussed in A. M. Garber, M. C. Weinstein, G. W. Torrance, and M. S. Kamlet in "Theoretical Foundations of Cost-effectiveness Analysis," in *Cost-effectiveness in Health and Medicine*, M. R. Gold et al., eds. (New York: Oxford University Press, 1996), pp. 25–53.

41. See Burton A. Weisbrod, "The Health Care Quadrilemma: An Essay on Technological Change, Insurance, Quality of Care, and Cost Containment," *Journal of Economic Literature*, Vol. 29 (June 1991), pp. 523–52. Joseph Newhouse has expressed some doubts about the insurance incentives in "Medical Care Costs: How Much Welfare Loss?" *Journal of Economic Perspectives*, Vol. 6 (Summer 1992), pp. 3–21.

42. Bryan R. Luce and Ruth E. Brown, "The Use of Technology Assessment by Hospitals, Health Maintenance Organizations, and Third-Party Payers in the United States," *International Journal of Technology Assessment in Health Care*, Vol. 11 (1995), pp. 79–92.

43. Richard A. Rettig has proposed a complementary, though somewhat more restrained (and thus perhaps more realistic) set of aims in "Medical Innovation Duels Cost Containment," *Health Affairs*, Vol. 13 (Summer 1994), pp. 8–27.

44. The setting of priorities is well argued in Auretine Gelijns and Nathan Rosenberg, "The Dynamics of Technological Change in Medicine," *Health Affairs*, Vol. 13 (Summer 1994), pp. 28–45.

FOUR: TWO-FACED NATURE: MEDICAL FRIEND OR MEDICAL FOE?

1. Quoted in Holmes Rolston III, *Philosophy Gone Wild: Essays in Environmental Ethics* (Buffalo: Prometheus Books, 1986), p. 6.

2. Quoted in George C. Williams, "Huxley's Evolution and Ethics in Sociobiological Perspective," *Zygon*, Vol. 23 (December 1988), p. 383.

3. F. H. Andersen, ed., *Francis Bacon: The New Organon and Related Writings* (Indianapolis: Bobbs-Merrill, 1960), p. 29. For a good

discussion of these issues, see Nancy S. Jecker, "Knowing When to Stop: The Limits of Nature," *Hastings Center Report*, Vol. 21 (May–June 1991), pp. 5–8.

4. Joseph Fletcher, *Morals and Medicine* (Princeton, N.J.: Princeton University Press, 1954), p. 11.

5. John Passmore, *Man's Responsibility for Nature: Ecological Problems and Western Traditions* (New York: Scribners, 1974), p. 187.

6. Carl Mitcham, "The Concept of Sustainable Development: Its Origins and Ambivalence," *Technology in Society*, Vol. 17 (1995), p. 314. Mitcham's essay is an excellent summary of the "sustainability" discussion and I have drawn on it liberally here.

7. International Union for Conservation of Nature and Natural Resources, *World Conservation Strategy* (Gland, Switzerland: United Nations Environmental Programme, 1980), Section 1, Paragraph 5; World Commission on Environment and Development, *Our Common Future* (New York: Oxford University Press, 1987).

8. Lester Brown, *Building a Sustainable Society* (New York: W. W. Norton, 1981).

9. Mitcham, op. cit., p. 324.

10. Gifford Pinchot, *The Fight for Conservation* (New York: Doubleday, 1910), p. 45.

11. Mark Sagoff, "What Is Environmentalism?" Unpublished paper, n.d., p. 4.

12. Bryan G. Norton, personal communication, 1996.

13. Henk Verhoog, "Two Concepts of Sustainability," unpublished lecture given at a Hastings Center conference, "Economics, Public Health, and the Environment," Prague, Czech Republic, August 26–27, 1991.

14. Hippocrates, "Precepts," in *Ethics in Medicine: Historical Perspectives and Contemporary Concerns*, S. J. Reiser, A. J. Dyck, and William J. Curran, eds. (Cambridge, Mass.: MIT Press, 1976), p. 6.

15. Rolston, op. cit., pp. 46–47.

16. Brown, op. cit., p. 10.

17. See Herman E. Daly, "Introduction to the Steady-State Economy," in *A Survey of Ecological Economics*, Rajaram Kirshnan, Nathan M. Harris, and Neva R. Goodwin, eds. (Washington, D.C.: Island Press, 1995), pp. 116–21.

18. Herman E. Daly, "Allocation, Distribution, and Scale: Toward an Economics That Is Efficient, Just, and Sustainable," in Krishnan, op. cit., pp. 121–24. I find particularly apt, also, another passage from Daly's writings: "The major task of environmental macroeconomics is to . . . keep the weight, the absolute scale, of the economy from sinking our environmental ark" (p. 123). Can the scale of contemporary health care systems be kept from sinking the economics of which they are a part? Or—better, perhaps—be kept from making those economies list very badly, always taking on water?

303

FIVE: SELF, SOCIETY, AND SUFFERING

1. Oliver Wendell Holmes, *Currents and Counter-Currents in Medical Science* (Boston: Ticknor and Fields, 1861), pp. 7–8.

2. James E. Sabin and Norman Daniels, "Determining Medical Necessity in Mental Health Practice," *Hastings Center Report*, Vol. 24 (September–October 1994), pp. 5–13.

3. I have developed this argument at greater length in *The Troubled Dream of Life: In Search of a Peaceful Death* (New York: Simon & Schuster, 1993).

4. Sherwin B. Nuland, *How We Die: Reflections on Life's Final Chapter* (New York: Alfred A. Knopf, 1994), pp. 259–60.

5. The biomedical model is carefully described in L. Foss and K. Rothenberg, *The Second Medical Revolution: From Biomedicine to Infomedicine* (Boston: Shambhala Publications and Random House, 1987).

6. Christopher Boorse, "On the Distinction Between Disease and Illness," *Philosophy and Public Affairs*, Vol. 5 (Fall 1975), pp. 49–78.

7. George L. Engel, "The Need for a New Medical Model: A Challenge for Biomedicine," *Science*, Vol. 196 (1977), pp. 129–36; George L. Engel, "The Clinical Application of the Biopsychosocial Model," *American Journal of Psychiatry*, Vol. 137 (1980), pp. 535–44. There is a rich discussion of these issues in Kerr L. White, *The Task of Medicine: Dialogue at Wickenburg* (Menlo Park, Calif.: The Henry J. Kaiser Family Foundation, 1988).

8. George L. Engel, "How Much Longer Must Medicine's Science Be Bound by a Seventeenth Century World View?" in White, op. cit., p. 120.

9. R. G. Evans and G. L. Stoddard, "Producing Health, Consuming Health Care," in *Why Are Some People Healthy and Others Not? The Determinants of Population Health*, Robert G. Evans, Morris L. Barer, and Theodore R. Marmor, eds. (New York: Aldine de Gruyter, 1994), pp. 27–64.

10. Particularly illuminating on these issues is a unpublished paper by the political scientist J. Donald Moon, presented at a meeting of The Hastings Center, "Thin Selves/Rich Lives: On the Concept of the Self in Liberal Theory," 1986.

11. This view has been expressed by John Rawls in "Justice as Fairness: Political Not Metaphysical," *Philosophy and Public Affairs*, Vol. 14 (Summer 1985), pp. 224–51; and in *Political Liberalism* (New York: Columbia University Press, 1993). For an effort to work liberalism out of this narrow political and philosophical foundation, see William Galston, "Defending Liberalism," *The American Political Science Review*, Vol. 76 (September 1987), pp. 621–29.

12. The political scientist Michael Sandel has been particularly effective here. See his book *Democracy's Discontent: America in Search of a Public Philosophy* (Cambridge, Mass.: Harvard University Press, 1996).

13. Michael Walzer has offered some interesting, indirectly pertinent reflections on the liberalism-communitarianism debate in "The Idea of a Civil Society," *Dissent* (Spring 1991), pp. 293–304.

14. Deborah A. Stone, "Commentary: The Durability of Social Capital," *Journal of Health Politics, Policy and Law*, Vol. 20 (Fall 1995), pp. 689–94.

15. See also Hans-Martin Sass, "The New Triad: Responsibility, Solidarity and Subsidiarity," *The Journal of Medicine and Philosophy*, Vol. 20 (December 1995), pp. 587–94.

16. John Stuart Mill, *Utilitarianism* (Indianapolis: Bobbs-Merrill, 1971), p. 23.

17. Courtney S. Campbell, "The Ordeal and Meaning of Suffering," *Sunstone*, Vol. 18 (December 1995), p. 39.

SIX: PUBLIC HEALTH AND PERSONAL RESPONSIBILITY

1. The most comprehensive case for this perspective is to be found in *Why Are Some People Healthy and Others Not? The Determinants of the Health of Populations*, Robert G. Evans, Morris L. Barer, and Theodore R. Marmor, eds. (New York: Aldine de Gruyter, 1994). See also, in a slightly more skeptical vein, John P. Bunker, Deanna S. Gomby, Barbara H. Kehrer, *Pathways to Health: The Role of Social Factors* (Menlo Park, Calif.: The Henry J. Kaiser Family Foundation, 1989). There is an interesting exchange on "social factors" as disease determinants in Sylvia N. Tesh, "Miasma and 'Social Factors' in Disease Causality: Lessons from the Nineteenth Century," *Journal of Health Politics, Policy and Law*, Vol. 20 (Winter 1995), pp. 1000–1024, and Christopher Hamlin, "Finding a Function for Public Health: Disease Theory or Political Philosophy," *Journal of Health Politics, Policy and Law*, Vol. 20 (Winter 1995), pp. 1025–1030; Bruce Link and Jo C. Phelan, "Editorial: Understanding Sociodemographic Differences in Health—The Role of Fundamental Social Causes," *American Journal of Public Health*, Vol. 86 (April 1996), pp. 471–72. A particularly helpful article is Constance A. Nathanson, "Disease Prevention as Social Change: Toward a Theory of Public Health," *Population and Development Review*, Vol. 22 (December 1996), pp. 609–637.

2. See Larry Gordon, "Public Health Is More Important Than Health Care," *Journal of Public Health Policy*, Vol. 11 (1993), pp. 261–64.

3. U.S. Department of Health and Human Services, *For a Healthy Nation: Returns on Investment in Public Health* (Washington, D.C.: U.S. Government Printing Office, 1994); see also John K. Iglehart, "Politics and Public Health," *The New England Journal of Medicine*, Vol. 234 (January 18, 1996), pp. 203–207. Paul Starr has written interestingly on the travails and decline of public health in the late nineteenth century, resisted by physicians, religious groups, and business: *The Transformation of American Medicine* (New York: Basic Books, 1982), pp. 180–97.

4. Institute of Medicine, *The Future of Public Health* (Washington, D.C.: National Academy Press, 1988); see also George J. Annas, "Back to the Future: The IOM Report Reconsidered," *America Journal of Public Health*, Vol. 81, No. 7 (July 1991), pp. 835–37.

5. *For a Healthy Nation*, op. cit., p. 4.

6. See Milton Terris, "Concepts of Health Promotion: Dualities in Public Health Theory," *Journal of Public Health Policy*, Autumn 1992, pp. 267–75.

7. Molly Joel Coye in *Leadership in Public Health*, Molly Joel Coye, William H. Foege, and William L. Roper (New York: Milbank Memorial Fund, 1994), p. 2.

8. Ibid., p. 5.

9. Robert W. Ambler and H. Bruce Dull, *Closing the Gap: The Burden of Unnecessary Illness* (New York: Oxford University Press, 1987); and J. Michael McGinnis and William Foege, "Actual Causes of Death in the United States," *Journal of the American Medical Association*, Vol. 270 (November 10, 1993), pp. 2207–2212.

10. This position is put forward, in a most lively way, by Peter Skrabanek, *The Death of Humane Medicine and the Rise of Coercive Healthism* (London: The Social Affairs Unit, 1994); see also Marshall H. Becker, "The Tyranny of Health Promotion," *Public Health Review*, Vol. 14 (1986), pp. 15–25.

11. Charles J. Dougherty, "Bad Faith and Victim-Blaming: The Limits of Health Promotion," *Health Care Analysis*, 1993, pp. 111–19; Arthur Caplan, "Sinners, Saints, and Health Care: Personal Responsibility and Health Care," *Northwest Report*, Vol. 24 (April 1994), pp. 20–23; Dan Wikler, "Who Should Be Blamed for Being Sick?" *Health Education Quarterly*, Vol. 14 (Spring 1987), pp. 11–25.

12. For a good discussion of the causal issue, see Alan M. Garber, "Pursuing the Links Between Socioeconomic Factors and Health: Critique, Policy Implications, and Directions for Future Research," in Bunker, Gomby, and Kehrer, op. cit., pp. 271–315; Ann Robertson and Meredith Minkler, "New Health Promotion Movement: A Critical Examination," *Health Education Quarterly*, Vol. 21 (Fall 1994), pp. 295–312.

NOTES

13. Paul M. Ellwood, Jr., and George D. Lundberg, "Managed Care: A Work in Progress," *Journal of the American Medical Association,* Vol. 276 (October 2, 1996), pp. 1083–1086; Thomas Bodenheimer, "The HMO Backlash—Righteous or Reactionary," *The New England Journal of Medicine,* Vol. 335 (November 21, 1996), pp. 1601–1603; Ronald Ray Loeppke, "Prevention and Managed Care: The Next Generation," *Journal of Occupational and Environmental Medicine,* Vol. 37 (May 1995), pp. 558–62; Helen Halpin Schauffler and Tracy Rodriguez, "Managed Care for Preventive Services: A Review of Policy Options," *Medical Care Review,* Vol. 50 (Summer 1993), pp. 153–98; Centers for Disease Control and Prevention, "Prevention and Managed Care: Opportunities for Managed Care Organizations, Purchasers of Health Care, and Public Health Agencies," *Morbidity and Mortality Weekly Report,* Vol. 44 (November 17, 1995), pp. 1–12.

14. Gerald Dworkin, "Taking Risks, Assessing Responsibility," *Hastings Center Report,* Vol. 11 (October 1981), p. 31.

15. Richard H. Nicholson, "U.K. Moves Toward Compulsory Vaccination," *Hastings Center Report,* Vol. 26 (March–April 1996), p. 4.

16. John Powles, "On the Limitations of Modern Medicine," *Science, Medicine & Man,* Vol. 1 (1973), p. 24.

17. U.S. Department of Health and Human Services, *For a Healthy Nation,* op. cit. Lester Breslow's writings have most decisively demonstrated the health benefits of a salubrious way of life. See, for instance, "Health Practices and Disability: Some Evidence from Alameda County," *Preventive Medicine,* Vol. 22 (1993), pp. 86–95. See also Richard G. Rogers, "Sociodemographic Characteristics of Long-Lived and Healthy Individuals," *Population and Development Review,* Vol. 21 (March 1995) pp. 33–58.

18. It is not difficult to find any number of statements and claims about the benefits of health promotion and disease prevention. See Phyllis Freeman and Anthony Robbins, "National Health Care Reform Minus Public Health: A Formula for Failure," *Journal of Public Health Policy,* Vol. 15 (Autumn 1994); U.S. Department of Health and Human Services, *For a Healthy Nation,* op. cit.; U.S. Department of Health and Human Services, "An Ounce of Prevention: What Are the Returns?" (Atlanta Centers for Disease Control and Prevention, n.d. [circa 1994]); The World Bank, *World Development Report 1993* (New York: Oxford University Press, 1993), p. 8; James W. Henderson, "The Cost Effectiveness of Prenatal Care," *Health Care Financing Review,* Vol. 15 (Summer 1994), pp. 21–32; James F. Fries et al., "Reducing Health Care Costs by Reducing the Need and Demand for Medical Services," *The New England Journal of Medicine,* Vol. 329 (July 29, 1993), pp. 321–25. Other analysts are more cautious, however, most notably the economist Louise Russell. Responding to the article by Fries and his co-

authors, Russell wrote: "The cost-effectiveness of many preventive services has yet to be evaluated in good studies. Until it is, it would be premature to conclude that such services will reduce medical expenditures. . . . Many preventive services do not save money, but some are good values nonetheless, when compared with other uses of the health care dollar." *The New England Journal of Medicine*, Vol. 329 (July 29, 1993), pp. 353–54. For some arguments in the same vein, see C. Patterson and Larry W. Chambers, "Preventive Health Care," *The Lancet*, Vol. 345 (June 24, 1995), p. 1614; and David Stipp, "Prevention May Be Costlier Than a Cure," *The Wall Street Journal*, July 6, 1994, p. 1, reporting on a study carried out by the Harvard School of Public Health's Center for Risk Analysis. Kenneth Warner, analyzing the implications of a tobacco-free society, concluded: "The economic implications of a tobacco-free society would be modest and of far less consequence than the principal implication: a significantly enriched quality and quantity of life" (*Journal of the American Medical Association*, Vol. 258 [October 16, 1987], pp. 2081–2086). Finally, see Anne Glixhauser (guest editor), "Health Care Cost-Benefit and Cost Effectiveness Analysis (CBA/CEA): From 1979–1990: A Bibliography," *Medical Care*, Supplement 31 (July 1993).

19. See, especially, Willard Gaylin and Bruce Jennings, *The Proper Use of Coercion and Constraints in a Free Society* (New York: The Free Press, 1996).

20. Martha Perske, "Are Anti-Smokers Attempting to Manipulate the Public?" *The NSA [National Smokers Alliance] Voice*, Vol. 4 (March 1996), pp. 1–3.

21. Daniel I. Wikler, "Persuasion and Coercion for Health: Ethical Issues in Government Efforts to Change Life-Styles," *Milbank Memorial Fund Quarterly*, Vol. 56 (1978), pp. 303–338.

22. Haavi Morreim, "Lifestyles of the Risky and Infamous: From Managed Care to Managed Lives," *Hastings Center Report*, Vol. 25 (November–December 1995), p. 65. See also Brian Smart, "Fault and the Allocation of Spare Organs," *Journal of Medical Ethics*, Vol. 20 (1994), pp. 26–30.

23. George J. Annas, personal communication, 1996.

24. Faith T. Fitzgerald, "The Tyranny of Health," *The New England Journal of Medicine*, Vol. 331 (July 21, 1994), p. 197.

25. James L. Nichols, "Changing Public Behavior for Better Health: Is Education Enough?" in "Medicine in the Twenty-first Century: Challenges in Personal and Public Health Promotion," *American Journal of Preventive Medicine*, supplement to Vol. 10 (May–June 1994), pp. 19–22.

26. Meredith Minkler, "Practitioners' Forum," *American Journal of Health Promotion*, Vol. 8 (July–August 1994), p. 405. See also Jonathan

Mann, "Human Rights and the New Public Health," *Health and Human Rights*, Vol. 1 (1995), pp. 229–33.

27. T. R. Marmor, M. L. Barer, and R. G. Evans, "The Determinants of a Population's Health: What Can Be Done to Improve a Democratic Nation's Health Status?" in Evans, Barer, and Marmor, eds., op. cit., pp. 223–24.

28. Robert P. Heaney, "The Intersalt Study Reveals Some Unexpected Connections," *America* (May 4, 1996), p. 20.

29. Some useful research strategies are outlined in Neil Pearce, "Traditional Epidemiology, Modern Epidemiology, and Public Health," *American Journal of Public Health*, Vol. 86 (May 1996), pp. 678–83.

30. My approach is narrower than that taken by the Swedish health philosopher Lennart Nordenfelt in *Toward a Theory of Health Promotion: A Logical Analysis* (Health Service Studies 5, Linkoping Collaborating Centre—LCC [Linkoping, Sweden: Linkoping University, 1991]).

31. David Mechanic, "An Examination of Underlying Processes," in Bunker, Gomby, and Kehrer, op. cit., pp. 9–26.

32. Jeffrey P. Kaplan and John R. Livengood, "The Influence of Changing Demographic Patterns on Our Health Promotion Priorities," in "Medicine in the Twenty-first Century: Challenges in Personal and Public Health Promotion," op. cit., pp. 42–44.

33. A harbinger of what I have in mind was reported in a *Wall Street Journal* story (June 30, 1997, p. 1). It reported, of managed care, that "There are hints it may be slowing the costly medical technology, slowing cost increases but raising uncomfortable questions." The "uncomfortable questions" concern the likely impact of such a trend, if that's what it is, on the development of new technologies and on the quality of care. From my perspective, that is a comforting prospect; we can stand a reduction in that quality of care that requires ever new technologies and in the supposed imperative to constantly develop new technologies. "The march of managed care," the story concludes, "may be the mechanism for slowing the advance of expensive medical technology. If so, what looked like a temporary lull in health care costs could be a significantly longer-lasting phenomenon."

SEVEN: CAN THIS MARRIAGE SUCCEED? MEDICINE AND THE MARKET

1. Perhaps the most important market proponent allowing a significant role for government is the Stanford management professor Alain Enthoven. His efforts, together with Paul M. Ellwood, as part of what came to be called the Jackson Hole Group have aimed to find ways to improve the working of the market with the ultimate goal of "adequate

health protection for everyone." See Paul M. Ellwood and Alain C. Enthoven, "'Responsible Choices': The Jackson Hole Group Plan for Health Reform," *Health Affairs*, Vol. 14 (Summer 1995), pp. 24–39. See also Alain Enthoven and Richard Kronick, "A Consumer Health-Choice Plan for the 1990s: Universal Health Insurance in a System Designed to Promote Quality and Economy," *The New England Journal of Medicine*, Vol. 320 (January 5, 1989), pp. 29–37. A most effective critique of the role of the market in medicine is to be found in Robert Kuttner, *Everything for Sale: The Virtues and Limits of Markets* (New York: Alfred A. Knopf, 1997), especially Chapter 4, "Market and Medicine," pp. 110–58.

2. Plato, *The Republic*, trans. F. M. Cornford, *The Works of Plato* (Oxford, England: Oxford University Press, 1945), pp. 22–24.

3. Adam Smith, *Wealth of Nations* (Buffalo: Prometheus Books, 1991), p. 20.

4. C. P. Snow, *The Two Cultures and the Scientific Revolution* (Cambridge, England: Cambridge University Press, 1993).

5. The most impassioned opponent of medicine's turn to the market is Dr. Arnold S. Relman, editor emeritus of *The New England Journal of Medicine*. See in particular "What Market Values Are Doing to Medicine," *The Atlantic Monthly*, Vol. 269 (March 1992), pp. 98–106. A less anxious view is that of David Blumenthal, "Effects of Market Reform on Doctors and Their Patients," *Health Affairs*, Vol. 15 (Summer 1996), pp. 170–84; considerably more neutrality is displayed in Wynand P. M. M. Van De Ven, "Market-Oriented Health Care Reforms: Trends and Future Options," *Social Science and Medicine*, Vol. 43 (1996), pp. 655–66.

6. Christopher Pass et al., *The HarperCollins Dictionary of Economics* (New York: HarperCollins, 1991), p. 321. See also Bernard Barber, "All Economies Are 'Embedded': The Career of a Concept, and Beyond," *Social Research*, Vol. 62 (Summer 1995), pp.387–413, for an insightful analysis of the history and use of the term "market."

7. James A. Morone and Janice M. Goggin, "Health Policies in Europe: Welfare States in a Market Era," *Journal of Health Politics, Policy and Law*, Vol. 20 (Fall 1995), pp. 557–69; see also Regina E. Herzlinger, *Market-Driven Health Care: Who Wins, Who Loses in the Transformation of America's Largest Service Industry?* (Reading, Mass.: Addison-Wesley, 1997), and Richard A. Epstein, *Mortal Peril: Our Inalienable Right to Health Care?* (Reading, Mass.: Addison-Wesley, 1997), both of whom argue for the economic and humanitarian benefits of the market in health care.

8. Maurizio Ferrara, "The Rise and Fall of Democratic Universalism: Health Care Reform in Italy, 1978–1994," *Journal of Health Politics, Policy and Law*, Vol. 20 (Summer 1995), pp. 275–302.

9. Daniel Sarewitz, *Frontiers of Illusion: Science, Technology, and the Politics of Progress* (Philadelphia: Temple University Press, 1996), p. 119.

10. Amartya Sen, *On Ethics and Economics* (Oxford, England: Blackwell Publishers, 1987), p. 28.

11. Alan Wolfe, *Whose Keeper: Social Science and Moral Imagination* (Berkeley: University of California Press, 1989), pp. 29–30.

12. Smith, op. cit., p. 46. See also Emma Rothschild, "Adam Smith and Conservative Economics," *Economic History Review*, Vol. 45 (1992), pp. 74–96.

13. Gary S. Becker, *The Economic Approach to Human Behavior* (Chicago: University of Chicago Press, 1976), p. 5.

14. George J. Stigler, *The Economist as Preacher and Other Essays* (Chicago: University of Chicago Press, 1982), p. 35.

15. Robert G. Royce, "Observations on the NHS Internal Market: Will the Dodo Get the Last Laugh?" *British Medical Journal*, Vol. 310 (August 12, 1995), pp. 431–33; Alan Maynard, "Competition in the UK National Health Service: Mission Impossible?" *Health Policy*, Vol. 23 (1993), pp. 193–204; Alan Maynard and Karen Bloor, "Introducing a Market to the United Kingdom's National Health Service," *The New England Journal of Medicine*, Vol. 334 (February 29, 1996), pp. 604–607.

16. Donald E. Frey, "The Good Samaritan as Bad Economist: Self-Interest in Economics and Theology," *Cross Currents* (Fall 1996), pp. 301–302.

17. See Edmund C. Pellegrino and David C. Thomasma, *For the Patient's Good: The Restoration of Beneficence in Health Care* (New York: Oxford University Press, 1988).

18. "America Then and Now," *Time* (January 29, 1996), p. 38.

19. Lincoln C. Chen and Linda G. Hiebert, "From Socialism to Private Markets: Vietnam's Health in Rapid Transition," Working Paper Series Number 94.11, Harvard Center for Population and Development Studies (October 1994); William C. L. Hsiao, "The Chinese Health Care System: Lessons for Other Nations," *Social Science and Medicine*, Vol. 41 (1995), pp. 1047–1055; see also Nguyen Tran Hien et al., "The Pursuit of Equity: A Health Sector Case Study from Vietnam," *Health Policy*, Vol. 33 (1995), pp. 191–204.

20. Allen Buchanan, "Privatization and Just Healthcare," *Bioethics*, Vol. 9 (1995), pp. 220–39; see also Buchanan's earlier and most insightful book *Ethics, Efficiency and the Market* (Totowa, N.J.: Rowman and Allanheld, 1985).

21. Eli Ginsberg, "A Cautionary Note on Market Reforms in Health Care," *Journal of the American Medical Association*, Vol. 274 (November 22–29, 1995), pp. 1633–34.

22. James C. Robinson and Harold S. Luft, "Competition and the Cost of Hospital Care, 1972 to 1982," *Journal of the American Medical Association*, Vol. 257 (June 19, 1987), pp. 3241–45; James C. Robinson et al., "Hospital Competition and Surgical Length of Stay," *Journal of the American Medical Association*, Vol. 259 (February 5, 1988), pp. 696–700.

23. Burton A. Weisbrod, "Competition in Health Care: A Cautionary View," (Washington, D.C.: American Enterprise Institute, 1983), pp. 61–62.

24. Alan Maynard, "Can Competition Enhance Efficiency in Health Care? Lessons from the Reform of the U.K. National Health Service," *Social Science and Medicine*, Vol. 39 (1994), p. 1433; a more optimistic view is presented in Alain C. Enthoven and Sara J. Singer, "Managed Competition and California's Health Economy," *Health Affairs*, Vol. 15 (Spring 1996), pp. 39–55; Warren Greenberg, ed., *Competition in the Health Care Sector* (Germantown, Md.: Aspen Systems, 1978); see also Eli Ginzberg, "Managed Care and the Competitive System in Health Care," *Journal of the American Medical Association*, Vol. 277 (June 11, 1997), pp. 1812–13.

25. Joseph P. Newhouse, "Economists, Entrepreneurs, and Health Care Reform," *Health Affairs*, Vol. 14 (Spring 1995), p. 188.

26. Paul M. Ellwood, Jr., and George D. Lundberg, "Managed Care: A Work in Progress," *Journal of the American Medical Association*, Vol. 276 (October 2, 1996), pp. 1083–1086.

27. Paul T. Menzel, "Economic Competition in Health Care: A Moral Assessment," *The Journal of Medicine and Philosophy*, Vol. 12 (February 1987), pp. 63–84; see also George W. Rainbolt, "Competition and the Patient-Centered Ethic," *The Journal of Medicine and Philosophy*, Vol. 12 (February 1987), pp. 85–99; and Ronald C. Lippincott and James W. Begun, "Competition in the Health Sector: A Historical Perspective," *Journal of Health Politics, Policy and Law*, Vol. 7 (Summer 1982), pp. 460–87.

28. Alan Wolfe's discussion, "Markets and Intimate Obligations," in Wolfe, op. cit., pp. 51–77, is particularly illuminating here.

29. The high-water mark of a "right" to health care was apparently reached in the early 1980s, with a significant decline thereafter in the invocation of that phrase. See James F. Childress, "Rights to Health Care in a Democratic Society," in *Biomedical Ethics Review, 1984*, James M. Humber and Robert Almeder, eds. (Clifton, N.J.: Humana Press, 1984), pp. 47–71; and "Rights to Health Care," a special issue of *The Journal of Medicine and Philosophy*, Vol. 4 (June 1979).

30. See, for instance, the writings of Norman Daniels, especially *Just Health Care* (Cambridge, England: Cambridge University Press, 1985); Robert H. Blank, *The Price of Life: The Future of American Health Care* (New York: Columbia University Press, 1997).

31. President's Commission for the Study of Ethical Problems in Medicine and Biomedical and Behavioral Research, *Securing Access to Health Care*, Vol. 1 (Washington, D.C.: U.S. Government Printing Office, 1983), p. 22.

32. This issue is well analyzed by Elizabeth Anderson, *Value in Ethics and Economics* (Cambridge, Mass.: Harvard University Press, 1993), especially in Chapter 7. See also Julian Le Grand, "Markets and Quasi-Markets in Health Care," *Eurohealth*, Vol. 1 (October 1995), p. 3; Sara Bennett, "The Public/Private Mix in Health Care Systems," in *Health Policy and Systems Development*, Katja Janovsky, ed. (Geneva, Switzerland: World Health Organization, 1996), pp. 101–123.

33. Jerome P. Kassirer, "Managed Care and the Morality of the Marketplace," *The New England Journal of Medicine*, Vol. 333 (July 6, 1995), p. 50; see also David Orentlicher, "Paying Physicians to Do Less: Financial Incentives to Limit Care," *University of Richmond Law Review*, Vol. 30 (1996), pp. 155–97.

34. A negative assessment of cost sharing as an incentive to control costs has been argued by M. Edith Rasell, "Cost Sharing in Health Insurance—A Reexamination," *The New England Journal of Medicine*, Vol. 332 (April 27, 1995), pp. 1164–68. Rasell contends: "The negative benefits of policies intended to make consumers more cost conscious outweigh any likely benefits . . . global budgets, capital budgeting, negotiated rates, and expenditure caps [would be more effective]" (p. 1168). But it strikes me that those measures, to work, would entail patient cost-sharing. See also Richard B. Saltman and Joseph Figueras, "On Solidarity and Competition: An Evidence-Based Perspective," *Eurohealth*, Vol. 2 (December 1996), pp. 19–20. The authors agree that cost-sharing incentives for patients are not effective, while incentives to hold down costs for those who supply care are.

35. James Q. Wilson, "Capitalism and Morality," *The Public Interest*, Vol. 21 (Fall 1970), p. 60.

EIGHT: EQUITY AND A STEADY-STATE MEDICINE

1. Norman Daniels, Donald W. Light, Ronald L. Caplan, *Benchmarks of Fairness for Health Care Reform* (New York: Oxford University Press, 1996), p. 19; see also Norman Daniels, *Just Health Care* (Cambridge, England: Cambridge University Press, 1985); World Health Organization, *Renewing the Health-for-All Strategy* (Geneva, Switzerland: World Health Organization, 1995).

2. Robert G. Evans, "Health Care as a Threat to Health," *Daedalus* 123 (Fall 1994), pp. 21–42. See also John N. Lavis and Gregory L. Stoddart, "Can We Have Too Much Health Care?" *Daedalus*, Vol. 123 (Fall 1994), pp. 43–60.

3. The most comprehensive data on health care inequality can be found in U.S. Department of Health and Human Services, *Health United States 1994* (Washington, D.C.: National Center for Health Statistics, May 1995).

4. For an international analysis of inequalities, see Christopher J. L. Murray and Alan D. Lopez, eds., *The Global Burden of Disease* (Cambridge, Mass.: Harvard University Press, 1996), and The World Bank, *World Development Report 1993: Investing in Health* (New York: Oxford University Press, 1993). An important article bearing more broadly on equity and health is Richard G. Wilkinson, "The Epidemiological Transition: From Material Scarcity to Social Disadvantage," *Daedalus*, Vol. 123 (Fall 1994), pp. 61–77. Wilkinson shows that it is not per capita income growth that solely affects mortality rates but, instead, "the inequality of income in each society" (p. 61).

5. René Dubos, *Mirage of Health* (New York: Harper & Row, 1959).

6. Cited in Rick J. Carlson, *The End of Medicine* (New York: John Wiley & Sons, 1995), p. 62.

7. Kevin Grumbach and Thomas Bodenheimer, "Painful vs. Painless Cost Control," *Journal of the American Medical Association*, Vol. 272 (November 9, 1994); David M. Eddy, "Benefit Language: Criteria That Will Improve Quality While Reducing Costs," *Journal of the American Medical Association*, Vol. 275 (February 28, 1996), pp. 650–57.

8. Victor R. Fuchs, "No Pain, No Gain: Perspectives on Cost Containment," *Journal of the American Medical Association*, Vol. 269 (February 3, 1993), pp. 631–33; David M. Eddy, "Health System Reform: Will Controlling Costs Require Rationing Services?" *Journal of the American Medical Association*, Vol. 272 (July 27, 1994), pp. 324–28; Richard Smith, "Rationing Health Care: Moving the Debate Forward," *British Medical Journal*, Vol. 312 (June 22, 1996), pp. 1553–54; Health Policy and Economic Research Unit, *British Medical Journal*, "Rationing Revisited: A Discussion Paper," Discussion Paper No. 4 (June 1995).

9. In their study of the "global burden of disease," the public health physicians Christopher Murray and Alan Lopez noted that "a range of studies confirms [a] broad social preference to 'weight' the value of a year lived by a young adult more heavily than one lived by a very young child or an older adult." Christopher J. L. Murray and Alan D. Lopez, *Summary: The Global Burden of Disease* (Geneva, Switzerland: World Health Organization, 1996), p. 9.

10. The dire projections for the American Medicare program have a European counterpart: "Europe Faces a Grey Future," *The Guardian* (London), April 3, 1996, p. 2.

11. Anne A. Scitovsky, "The High Cost of Dying: What Do the Data Show?" *Milbank Memorial Fund Quarterly*, Vol. 62 (Fall 1984), pp. 606–607. These figures have remained remarkably stable in the last decade.

12. I have developed this point at greater length in *The Troubled Dream of Life: In Search of a Peaceful Death* (New York: Simon & Schuster, 1993).

13. Anita F. Sarro, "Determining Medical Necessity Within Medicaid: A Proposal for Statutory Reform," *Nebraska Law Review*, Vol. 8 (1984), pp. 835, 842–43.

14. See Rudolf Klein, *The Politics of the National Health Service* (London: Longman, 1985).

15. United States Bipartisan Commission on Comprehensive Health Care, *A Call for Action* (Washington, D.C.: U.S. Government Printing Office, 1990), pp. 61–63.

16. David C. Hadorn, "Defining Basic Health Benefits Using Clinical Guidelines" (unpublished paper, 1994).

17. David M. Eddy, "What Care Is 'Essential'? What Services Are 'Basic'?" *Journal of the American Medical Association*, Vol. 256 (February 13, 1991), p. 782.

18. Ibid., p. 788.

19. John Immerwahr and Jean Johnson, *Second Opinions: Americans' Changing Views on Health Care Reform* (New York: The Public Agenda Foundation, 1994).

20. Klein, op. cit., p. 165.

21. See Ralph L. Keeney, "Decisions About Life-Threatening Risks," *The New England Journal of Medicine*, Vol. 331 (July 21, 1994), pp. 193–96.

Index

political dimension of,
261–62, 265
priorities in, 270–71
service-oriented approach to,
263–64
sustainability and, 260–61
U.S. vs. European systems
and, 262–63
Health and Human Services
Department, U.S., 177
public health as defined by,
178–79
Health Care and Financing Administration, 33
Health Care Technology Institute, 85, 86
health insurance, 13, 224, 225,
266
in Europe, 269
Health Insurance Association of
America, 94
health maintenance organizations (HMOs), 18, 117,
188
health promotion by, 177,
182
heart disease, 26, 65–66, 136,
182, 244, 247, 256, 278
Hippocrates, 21, 247
Hippocratic Oath, 214
History of the Idea of Progress
(Nisbet), 53–54
HIV disease, 64–65, 91, 183,
282
holistic medicine, 117
Holmes, Oliver Wendell, 139
Holton, Gerald, 52
homeopathic medicine, 117–18
Huxley, T. H., 113–14, 145
hygeia, tradition of, 22, 125,
175, 276

aesculapius vs., 42, 112,
173–74
nature and, 127, 128

Idea of Progress, The (Bury), 52
Illich, Ivan, 17, 18
infant mortality, 61, 63, 105,
133, 225, 242–43, 244
infectious disease, 64–65, 73,
118, 129, 285
infertility, 253–54
influenza, 64
Intersalt study, 202
Investing in Health (World
Bank), 14–15

James, William, 113, 114
Japan, 75
Joyce, James, 54

Kassirer, Jerome P., 236
Kennedy, John F., 240
Kierkegaard, Søren, 54
Klima, Ivan, 55
Knowles, John, 37

Lappé, Marc, 65
Lasch, Christopher, 53, 55–56,
100
liberalism:
communitarianism vs.,
160–62, 163
market and, 220
life-cycle perspective, 136, 137,
138
adulthood and, 255–56
aging and, 115, 132–34,
256–57
birth and, 253–55
childhood and, 253–55
death, dying and, 257–58

321